PHANTASTICA

PHANTASTICA

A Classic Survey on the Use
and Abuse of Mind-Altering Plants

LOUIS LEWIN, M. D.

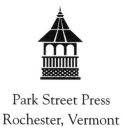

Park Street Press
Rochester, Vermont

Park Street Press
One Park Street
Rochester, Vermont 05767
www.gotoit.com

LIBRARY OF CONGRESS CATALOGING-IN-PUBLICATION DATA
Lewin, Louis, 1850–1929.
    [Phantastica.   English]
    Phantastica : a classic survey on the use and abuse of mind-altering plants /
        Louis Lewin.
      p. cm.
    Translated from the second German edition by P. H. A. Wirth.
    Includes index.
    ISBN 0-89281-783-6 (pbk. : alk. paper)
    1. Drugs of abuse. 2. Psychotropic plants. 3. Ethnobotany. I. Title.
    RM316.L4813   1998   98-9484
    615'.78—dc21   CIP

Printed and bound in Canada

10 9 8 7 6 5 4 3 2 1

Text design and layout by Rachel Goldenberg
This book was typeset in Goudy with Panache as the display typeface

Park Street Press is a division of Inner Traditions International

Distributed to the book trade in Canada by Publishers Group West (PGW),
    Toronto
Distributed to the book trade in the United Kingdom by Deep Books, London
Distributed to the book trade in Australia by Gemcraft Books, Burwood
Distributed to the book trade in New Zealand by Tandem Press, Auckland
Distributed to the book trade in South Africa by Alternative Books, Ferndale

CONTENTS

FOREWORD

With the present great interest in psychopharmacology it is only appropriate that a book like Louis Lewin's *Phantastica: Narcotic and Stimulating Drugs*, should be reprinted. The book was first published in German in 1924; the second German edition appeared in 1927, Italian and French translations in 1928 and the English version, now being reprinted in 1931. For more than 30 years the book has been a collectors' item.

By phantastica the author meant drugs giving rise to sense illusion, a much better word than the now commonly used name hallucinogenes, since most of these drugs do not give rise to true hallucinations but to distortions of perception. Phantastica, although only one group of the many compounds described in the book, has also been chosen as the name of the whole book, however, many other compounds like cocoa and tobacco are also included.

Louis Lewin's biography still remains to be written, but the reader of this book might benefit from a short presentation of his life and works, especially with regard to his achievements in psychopharmacology.

Louis Lewin was born in 1850 in the small town of Tuchel in Western Prussia. In 1854 he came to Berlin where he remained more or less until the end of his life. He graduated from the University of Berlin in 1875 as an M.D., studied for a while with Pettenkoffer and Voit in Munich, and became "Privatdozent" in pharmacology in Berlin in 1881. In 1894 he became titular professor at the University of Berlin but held no full academic position. Only as late as 1919 did he become permanent honorary professor at the Technical Academy. There has been much speculation about the reason why Lewin did not advance academically in pharmacology and toxicology and it has been said that he could have become head of the greatest pharmacology department in Germany had he renounced his Jewish faith and consented to become baptized. Whatever truth there may be in this, he established his

own private laboratory and lecture hall in Ziegelstrasse in an old tene-
ment house in the center of the medical district of Berlin. He preferred
to teach and to do his research with his own means in these surroundings. Financially he was partly enabled to do so through the fact that
although he had no official position, the courts preferred him to all
other experts in Germany in toxicology and industrial hygiene.

Lewin's way of lecturing was extraordinary and held the audiences
spellbound. It has been said that he expounded facts with a contagious enthusiasm and performed his little experiments with loving
care. Behind each of his sentences there was such deep faith in science and such unlimited devotion for the search for truth that nobody could remain indifferent. Any narrow specialization was foreign
to him. He could quote flawlessly in foreign languages without any
hesitation and marshal facts from all four corners of the world and all
periods of history. It will be apparent to the readers of *Phantastica* that
classical and contemporary authors were all familiar to him. He was a
great and strong personality, but he always worked alone; he had many
pupils but no assistants. He was, however, not only a lecturer but a
friend and advisor to his students with whom he often corresponded
afterwards for long periods of time and whom he sometimes helped to
the limit of his knowledge.

Many famous men who visited his lectures were deeply influenced
by him. Lewin's outstandingly wide general knowledge meant that he
had many friends among scholars in other facilities. With some of
them he published important papers, notably with the famous explorer
G. Schweinfurth and A. Miethe who were his good friends and who
esteemed him highly. In history, geography and anthropology his
knowledge was enormous; he showed special interest in travel and
topography and it is said that scarcely a travel book of importance was
unknown to him. His own traveling included visits, among other
places, to the United States, Switzerland and Italy.

His attitude towards art was also typical of this extraordinary man.
Here he combined appreciation of the classic works of art with manual
dexterity of his own. One of his pupils has recalled how in the intervals between lectures one could see him chase bronzes in a small room
next to the lecture hall. In 1901 he gave a lecture in the Archaeologi-
cal Society about the technique of antique bronzes.

When surveying Lewin's works one is greatly helped by a list he compiled himself before his death. The list includes 248 major publications in the years 1874–1929. From the list are excluded book reviews, printed discussions and other minor communications of his which were numerous. Among the publications there are about 12 books and monographs. Lewin himself claimed that by 1880 he had already decided to devote most of his time to the side effects of drugs. Also his first major work which appeared in 1881 *Nebenwirkungen der Arzneimittel* Pharmakologisch-klin. Handbuch. (Berlin: A. Hirschwald) dealt with this topic and became a classic and the first of its kind. This book had two more editions and was translated into three languages, including English. Notable among the other books are his outstanding textbook in toxicology, a summary of all available knowledge of arrow poisons, two volumes on the effect of drugs on the eye and another work in which he gives the world's history as seen by a toxicologist, *Die Gifte in der Weltgeschichte*, (Berlin: J. Springer, 1920).

It is not possible here to summarize all the fields of interest to which Lewin made original contributions, but it is appropriate to dwell on his activities in psychopharmacology, a topic in which he published some 20 books and papers. His own contributions to the fields occur mostly in the 1880s. Then he more or less left this field but in 1924 summarized admirably his own work and those of others in the first edition of the present book. The long delay certainly did not mean that he remained unfamiliar with the progress in the field; on the contrary, the books show that he kept up to date with all achievements made in the meantime.

Lewin's first publication, in 1874, was a study of chronic morphinism, which he was one of the first to investigate scientifically. In 1886 appeared his monograph on *Piper mythysticum* (Kawa Kawa): *Uber Piper methysticum* (Kawa Kawa). (Berlin: A. Hirschwald) a very comprehensive review of all aspects of the use of *Piper methysticum* and current research on its constituents and their chemistry, pharmacology and clinical effects. This admirable monograph is now understandably much out of date in its chemistry and pharmacology, but it was a pioneering work, and the period following its appearance saw the first real progress being made in the chemistry of the constituents of *Piper methysticum*.

In 1889 appeared another similar monograph: *Uber Areca Catechu, Chavica Betle und das Betelkauen*. (Stuttgart: F. Enke) an equally comprehensive review. Before that, however, Lewin had embarked upon a work to which he was going to revert many times during subsequent years. In 1886 he made a cross-country trip in the United States studying all aspects of toxicology and anthropology during his travels. Through the pharmaceutical house, Parke Davis & Co., he came into the possession of the mezcal buttons or Peyotl, used by Mexican and North American Indians ceremonially to produce changes in the state of mind. Until then very little was known as to the nature and character of this drug. Hennings, of the Botanical Museum of Berlin, recognized it as a new species of *anhalonium*, a view which has been challenged by other botanical specialists. In honor of Lewin he named it *"Anhalonium Lewinii."* In other works the cactus containing mescaline is referred to as *"Lophophorra Williamsii."* Lewin's first examination of the plant proved that it contained alkaloid substances, especially a crystallized alkaloid called by him anhalonine which had like the plant itself extremely strong exciting properties and which was capable of provoking muscular cramps in animals. The author himself admits that as a result of the experiments, nothing was learned of the process of excitation in the sensitive and sensorial sphere, but it was proved for the first time that there was in the family of the cacti hitherto regarded as biologically harmless a species possessing considerable and general toxic properties.

This discovery and others which followed excited a lively interest in the application of the drug in man. Thus Arthur Heffter (1860–1925) succeeded in isolating a series of chemically pure alkaloids. He studied these compounds pharmacologically both in animals and in heroic experiments on himself, by which he found out that mescaline was the psychopharmacologically active alkaloid. Lewin's friend Kurt Behringer later carried out numerous experiments in man with mescaline which resulted in a much-read monograph. The interest in the active principle first demonstrated by Lewin in the cactus has remained up to the present day and may even be said to have increased in recent years. It can be said that from 1890 to 1924 *"Anhalonium Lewinii"* was the only topic in psychopharmacology to which Lewin frequently came back to in his writings. It must have been one of his favorite observations even though he himself did not study the psychic effect in man.

A renewed interest in psychopharmacology was awakened in Lewin in 1928. In this year the 78-year-old research worker had a cerebral hemorrhage which partially paralyzed him but fortunately left his mental faculties intact. Through the devotion of his wife and friends he was nursed back to partial recovery and resumed his intellectual labours. It was at this time that he became interested in the properties of *Banisteria Caapi*, a South American plant said to be used for the treatment of senile paralysis. We now know that this plant contains alkaloids with monomine oxidase inhibiting properties and excitatory action on the nervous system. This was the last original contribution of Louis Lewin on psychopharmacology. His last work was to edit the 4th edition of his famous textbook on toxicology (which has recently been reprinted) *Gifte und Vergiftungen* (Karl F. Haug Verlag, Ulm/Donau), where the interested reader may look up all details and references to in the present book. Soon afterwards, at the age of 79 years, Louis Lewin died, described in an obituary by one of his pupils as: "Pharmacologist, toxicologist, medical historian, keen scientist, brilliant teacher, profound scholar, fascinating writer, a man of noble character, lofty ideals, and loyal to his race and faith."

Bo Holmstedt
Department of Pharmacology
Karolinska Institutet, Stockholm

PREFACE

Of the innumerable chemical substances other than foodstuffs which the world contains, none have a more intimate connection with human life than those whose history and effects are described in this work.

I have called it *Phantastica*, but this name which I have chosen does not cover all that I should wish it to convey. Nearly all the drugs dealt with have a direct action on the brain, an action which is in all its forms mysterious and incomprehensible.

If human consciousness is the most wonderful thing on earth, the attempt to fathom the depths of the psychophysiological action of narcotic and stimulating drugs makes this wonder seem greater still, for with their help man is enabled to transfer emotions of everyday life, as well as his will and intellect, to unknown regions; he is enabled to attain degrees of emotional intensity and duration which are otherwise unknown to the brain. Such effects are brought about by chemical substances. The most powerful of these are products of the vegetable kingdom, into whose silent growth and creative abundance man has not yet fully penetrated. By the exercise of their powers on the brain, they release marvelous stores of latent energy. They relieve the mentally tortured, assuage the racking pains of the sick, inspire with hope those doomed to death, endow the overworked with new vitality and vigour such as no strength of will could attain, and replace for an hour the exhaustion and languor of the overworked by mental comfort and content.

Miracles like these are performed throughout the world by these strange substances wherever men are in possession of any one of them. The savage in the jungle beneath a sheltering roof of leaves and the native of the storm-swept island secures through these drugs a greater intensity of life. The solitary dweller in a distant mountain cavern can with their aid relieve the dull monotony of his cramped existence. Various are the motives which induce civilized men to seek a transient sensation of pleasure. The potent influence of these substances leads us on the one hand into the darkest depths of human passion, ending in mental instability, physical misery, and degeneration, and on the other to hours of ecstasy and happiness or a tranquil and meditative state of mind.

Not only are these drugs of general interest to mankind as a whole, but they possess a high degree of scientific interest for the medical man, especially the psychologist and alienist, as well as for the jurist and ethnologist.

Varying degrees of mental susceptibility and vision, bordering upon mental disease, may result from an intemperate use of some of these substances. Hence arises for psycho-analytical science the possibility of analyzing more accurately certain mental phenomena which also occur in cases of insanity. A large field of activity and research is offered to psychology which hitherto was open only to a few scientific pioneers. The jurist needs an acquaintance with scientific facts bearing on the extent of the responsibility and soundness of judgment of those who, under the permanent influence of narcotic drugs come into collision with the civil or criminal law. To the ethnologist numerous problems, promising much new enlightenment, not to the least those relating to the study of comparative theology present themselves with regard to the extension and cause of the use of these drugs. The contents of this book will provide a starting-point from which original research in the above-mentioned departments of science may be pursued. I have avoided literary by-paths in order to follow more closely the direct line of pharmacological inquiry, but have nevertheless furnished the reader with a sufficiency of material and historical facts.

"There is hardly a more difficult chapter in the whole of pharmacology than an exhaustive and thoroughly exact analysis of the effects of drugs." These words, the view of a pharmacologist, are perfectly true. Since I published, in 1886, the first pharmacological and chemical report on one of these drugs, kava, which was made use of on a large scale, I have incessantly worked at these problems, and much of my work has been made public in subsequent volumes. The present book, the first of its kind, is meant not only to set forth the results of my pharmacological theories, which are supported by my own practical experience as well as by materials supplied by those who have come to me in search of help, but also to instruct and enlighten those who are endeavouring to see clearly amid the surging conflict of public opinion regarding drugs and the drug habit.

The first edition of this book having passed into many hands and received great praise, a second now appears, written with the same end in view but containing a greater volume of material.

The reader's attention is directed once more to the great problem set forth in these pages, a problem which cannot and will not be solved on the first attempt. Time is needed to produce that cure which is so desirable and necessary, for the enormous obstacles that bar the path of progress have deep roots in human passions; but every step directed to freeing men from such evils will prove a benefit to our race.

Louis Lewin

INTRODUCTION

General Remarks

From the first beginning of our knowledge of man, we find him consuming substances of no nutritive value, but taken for the sole purpose of producing for a certain time a feeling of contentment, ease, and comfort. Such a power was found in alcoholic beverages and in some vegetable substances, the same that are used for the purpose at the present day.

No chemical research has been able to produce synthetically anything in the slightest degree resembling the materials which peoples of all parts of the world have found suitable for their euphoric cravings. Their potential energy has conquered the whole earth and established communication between various races, in spite of dividing mountains and surrounding seas. These substances have formed a bond of union between men of opposite hemispheres, the uncivilized and the civilized; they have forced passages which, once open, proved of use for other purposes; they produced in ancient races characteristics which have endured to the present day, evidencing the marvelous degree of intercourse that existed between different peoples just as certainly and exactly as a chemist can judge the relation of two substances by their reactions. Hundreds or thousands of years were necessary to establish contact between whole nations by these means. Ethnology, which should endeavor to trace their routes, has never attempted to search out and investigate the elements of these questions, which are of equal importance to science and to the history of mankind. Careful inquiry, especially if combined with comparative linguistic studies, would unravel many such mysteries.

It is extremely important to note that the mere discovery of the properties and uses of narcotic and stimulating drugs implies a certain degree of scientific observation and marks the beginning of primeval

1

culture; and if it can be taken as a symptom of civilization when men's desires, hitherto exclusively confined to the bare necessities of life, pass beyond these limits, and the individual, no longer satisfied with the crude sustenance afforded by or wrested from nature, finds and delights in stimulants which mainly affect the nervous system, then a suitable background for such physical cravings must form part of the human constitution.

Motives for the Use of Narcotic and Stimulating Drugs

The motives for the occasional or habitual use of these drugs are of greater interest than collections of facts concerning them. Here all kinds of human contrasts meet; barbarism and civilization, with all their various degrees of material possessions, social status, knowledge, belief, age, gifts of body, mind, and soul.

On this plane meet artisan and sybarite, ruler and subject; the savage from some distant island or from the Kalahari desert associates with poets, philosophers, scientists, misanthropes, and philanthropists; the man of peace rubs shoulders with the man of war; the devotee with the atheist. The physical impulses which bring under their spell such diverse classes of mankind must be extraordinary and far-reaching. Many have expressed opinions about them but few have probed and understood their intrinsic properties, and fewer still perceived the innermost significance and the motives for the use of the substances in which such energies are stored.

It has been thought that the lower the position of a race on the ladder of mental capability, the cruder would be its preferred stimulants, and the more eagerly it would seek to deceive its earthly consciousness and to obtain deliverance from the emptiness of its inner life. The Indians of South America are said to have an intuitive appreciation of their own defectiveness, and to be ever ready to rid themselves of such melancholy feelings by intense excitement, i.e. through the use of kola and similar drugs.

Such men as Tolstoy, who were unable to comprehend these problems, even went so far as to assume that the reason for smoking and drinking is to dull the conscience, and the consumption of opium in the Malay Archipelago was due to "an insufficient education on a Christian basis." Such incredible absurdities are frequently to be met with. They are calculated on the one hand to excite surprise at the limited degree of observation of man and his passions possessed by those who hold them, and on the other they evoke an earnest desire to impart more knowledge on this subject to a larger public.

The strongest inducement to a frequent or daily use of the substances in question is to be found in the properties they posses; in their capacity to excite the functions of the brain-centres which transmit agreeable sensations and to maintain for sometime the consciousness of experienced emotions. Their results differ considerably. Even within the limits of either of the two large groups of possible effects, excitation and paralysis, their intensity of action varies extremely, adapting itself more or less adequately to the temporary condition of the nervous system of the user of the drug.

The inducements which bring about a first recourse to their use, especially in the case of narcotic substances, are just as varied. It may be mere curiosity which induces people to bring ridicule and harm upon themselves, or it may arise from a recognition of the drug's beneficial effect, after it has been taken during illness as a medicine; or again, it may result from the deliberate intention to effect a pleasant though temporary change in the state of the mind and soul, to divert the susceptibilities and thoughts into new channels. For instance, an Indian of Guatemala, asked why he drank so much aguardiente, answered: "A man must sometimes *zafarse de su memoria*," i.e. take a rest from his memory. It is an invariable rule that the remarkable properties possessed by these substances react on the brain and through it cause a craving for their habitual use and the accompanying pathological disturbances.

I have known men who first took a narcotic remedy from pure curiosity, and later, overcome by its influence, became habitual drug-takers. The publication in a popular form of scientific articles on the properties of these drugs has produced many cases of the drug habit. At the present time, when narcomania has reached an undreamed-of extent, even people who were incredulous as to the increase of this vice are astonished.

Well-known men have applied to me for a substance which, as they had been informed, brought about mental delusions and hallucinations. They hoped to experience agreeable sensations; one of them even meant to make use of such aid for poetical production, perhaps of a supernatural kind.

Many other circumstances could be mentioned which bring about the primary or continued use of narcotic and stimulating drugs. For life itself, and the life of the individual with its innumerable functional variations and idiosyncrasies, creates these strange causes which so often determine the normality, the decrepitude, or the annihilation of the individual.

The Importance of Mental Constitution in Relation to External Stimuli

The reasons for the habitual use of drugs, and the mental and physical results arising therefrom, have been accounted for in the preceding section by the peculiar effect which these drugs exercise on the brain. A number of problems, however, remain unexplained which likewise are of the utmost importance to the life of the individual: the varying reactions of different persons, not only to narcotics in general, but also to chemical and other influences, and the fact that one man can tolerate quantities, taken apparently with impunity within a short period, which to others would spell physical ruin. Indeed, the most elementary science teaches us that most drugs contain a high degree of latent energy which acts almost exclusively on the nervous system.

From time immemorial attempts have been made to solve these problems, but without success. Biology exerts its influence, and we enter on those deepest mysteries which man has ever endeavored to fathom: personality, mental constitution, and habit. Nothing thrusts itself more forcibly on our notice, nothing harasses the investigator more, nothing more prevents all deeper insight into this chaos of propositions and problems. They will always remain hidden from our view among the many disputable problems of life and vitality. We suffer, like Faust, from our inability to discover the truth, and must sincerely regret what Molière already satirically criticized: the fashion of clothing in meaningless Latin or Greek phrases what can never be known, or of repeating a mere surmise again and again until ignorant physicians or non-professional men venture to stamp it as a fundamental truth. Even to-day we frequently meet with interpretations of the action of medicinal and poisonous substances which are merely pseudo-scientific descriptions of their effects. We are reminded of the burlesque scene in Molière's *Le malade imaginaire* in which doctors of the University appear and examine a Bachelor of Medicine in a mixture

of Latin and French. Asked what is the ultimate reason for the soporific action of opium—

> *Demandabo causam et rationem quare*
> *Opium facit dormire,*

the candidate answers:

> *Quia est in eo*
> *Virtus dormitiva*
> *Cujus est natura*
> *Sensus assopire,*

i.e. "because it is endowed with narcotic and soporific properties,"
and the examiners call out in chorus:

> *Bene, bene, bene respondere*
> *Dignus, dignus est intrare*
> *In nostro docto copore.*

Unfortunately pharmacology and toxicology lend themselves with
particular ease to metaphysical absurdities of this description. These
doctrines are unable to withstand argument, and no enlightenment
can be expected from them. Drugs and poisons, with their potential
energies, are rooted in a material world which observes their active
properties but refuses to allow us to ask the reason for them.

Man's power of resistance to potent substances or his inability in
some cases to withstand them remain unexplained. The hypothesis
has been put forward that a distinct kind of energy exists which en-
velops and governs the whole of physical life. This we may call Vital
Energy. I include in this expression the sum of all the chemical, physical, and mechanical faculties which are dominated by the will but do
not respond to the same extent in all individual cases.

Every part of the body—brain, nerves, muscles, glands, intestines,
bones, or mucous membrane—every tissue, cellular or not, is provided
with this native energy. It is not that mystic power, *Spiritus rector* or
Archaeus, which played an important part in the theories of life of the
Middle Ages, but an organization of work which is, despite individual
dissimilarities, governed by manifest laws and immensely complicated
as it is, varies in strength and nature according to its location, destroying, building, dissolving, or strengthening as the case may be.

The amount of work actually depends on this factor.

Its active or passive manifestations show a greater or lesser degree of working or of toleration, non-toleration or varying toleration of external or internal influences of a stimulative or other nature. The appearance of these reactions varies to a great extent, even to the point of complete dissimilarity.

The impulse and ability to compensate for the disturbances caused by foreign bodies, should be included among these differences of organic life and their responses to material and other energies. Every organism has at its disposal a certain amount of prophylactic and regulating energy which varies in quantity, just as does the energy of the normal vital functions. I look upon this adaptable activity of prophylactic and defensive support as a reaction provided for the welfare of the individual and not as an innate necessity. I corroborate the opinion expressed by Pflüger in his *Teleological Mechanics:* "The cause of a desire in an organism is at the same time the source of the gratification of this desire," where by "cause of desire" is to be understood every alteration in the condition of the organism effected for the welfare of the individual. This self-defence always occurs to some extent, but ceases if, for instance, the chemically reactive power of a poison eliminates the vital energy either locally or over the whole body.

Perhaps it would be appropriate to refer to a consideration which has been for many years a subject of my lectures. It is conceivable that the impulse and the activity of regulating processes against foreign influences is enacted according to a scientific principle which has been termed by d'Alembert, Gauss, and later by Le Chatelier, the Law of Resistance to Constraint or the Law of Least Constraint, and which applies to chemical and physical processes. It may be thus stated: If to a system in equilibrium a constraint be applied, a change takes place within the system tending to nullify the effect of the constraint and to restore the equilibrium. The equilibrium is shifted in such a direction as will reduce the constraint. Systems in which the constraint applied is not reduced but magnified are not in a stable but in a labile equilibrium. In the human body both kinds exist. This is not the place to state in detail the consequences which the application of this principle to chemical reactions in the human body after the administration of a drug possess for scientific research. Enough to state that this new point of view will tend to facilitate our conception of many of the reactive phenomena of life.

Between the two possible extremes of the regulating of powers of the organism as a whole, success and failure, there are many intermediate stages, varying with the energy of the individual life. This for the most part hereditary factor, individual life, i.e. personal disposition, which does not show any apparent physical demeanor or difference in the tissue or humours of the body must be examined for every possible reactive influence. Human nature not only exists, but thrusts itself on our notice. To deny its great importance is a sign of medical ignorance, to underestimate it may be fatal, to explain its essence is impossible to mortal man. It is and always will remain in every respect a mystery. The attempt to bring forward the ductless glands as an explanation must be rejected because of its too limited interpretation of the personality. It constitutes an equation with so many unknown factors that its solution seems impossible.

It also causes individual differences in the normal corporal functions. Hardly any functions of the organs of the body, from the activity of the brain and the spinal cord to the work of the glands, the general metabolism, the movements of the internal organs, the development of muscular power, act to the same extent in different persons. These differences in physiological attainment must be placed on the same level as the result of external influences. From the most ancient times to the present day nothing has caused such astonishment among scientists and laymen as the fact that the causes of diseases, and also medicinal substances, whether poisonous or nourishing, produce such wholly diverse results both in human beings and in animals.

In the primeval history of mankind we are told that an injury which killed one man spared another, and that some animals could consume quantities of a poisonous plant which would cause the death of others or of man. Galen, that great medical genius, who, after being regarded as an authority for more than a thousand years, was discredited by those who did not know him, held pronounced views regarding the toleration of noxious substances and their habitual and occasional use, which are of greater value than many of the statements made to-day. The latter are, for the initiated, meaningless circumscriptions of the simple though inexplicable truth that the fluctuating

effective power which chemical substances have on certain individuals or races, has in like circumstances dissimilar effects on others, or is
neutralized by the peculiar constitution of some given individual. This
is true also of convalescence from sickness, wounds, or internal disorders. We may take it as a fact that Negroes have greater recuperation
powers than white people. This is due not to climatic conditions but
to certain innate qualities possessed by them.

Personal disposition affects every type of influence, mechanical,
chemical, or mental, and may be of an excessive or a sub-normal sensitivity or any degree between these extremes. A physically strong
man may be hypersensitive to a certain drug, a weak man hardly or
not at all affected by it. Personal disposition brings about the abnormal progress of toxic diseases as well as of those caused by narcotic
and stimulating drugs. None of them allow any prognosis. There is no
formula or rule which affords a definite standard, for general limits are
overpassed by the individual constitution.

As the astronomer has for his visual perception a "personal equation," so every man has probably what I would call a "toxic equation"—an expression first used by me and subsequently copied by dis-
honest plagiarists. By it I mean a greater or lesser sensibility of the
body or its organs to the effects of various chemical substances. It is
this toxic equation which causes a quantitative and sometimes a qualitative difference in functional reaction to one of these products. In
this case the inconceivable becomes a fact: for example, of two persons who are exposed in the same room to the toxic action of carbon
monoxide, one may be only slightly affected, whereas the other dies
or falls victim to some form of incurable cerebral disease, inflammation of the lungs, pulmonary gangrene, or some other disturbance of
the nutrition of the tissues. The transformation of the effective or
injurious influences into actual harm does not take place uniformly in
every human body. Until the present day no one has been able to
explain the real reason for this. It is one of the profound mysteries of
nature. The following words of Albrecht von Haller are and will always be applicable to these phenomena:

> Ins Innere der Natur[1]
> Dringt kein erschaffener Geist,
> Glückselig, wem sie nur
> Die aussere Schale weist.

Goethe, who lacked the authority of an expert, sought to refute his view. "For the poet," said he, "Nature has neither heart nor surface, to him she is both at once." Unfortunately, Haller's words are only too true. In biology, and in every sphere where nature affords problems of an unintelligible and inconceivable kind, there is indeed a heart and a surface; that which is visible and that which is concealed from our view. This is especially the case in biology; we recognize the dial of the clock and the movement of the hands, but we are unable to see the work and the driving power. We encounter the same unfathomable abyss as when we seek the origin of a living being, of one of its tissues or even but one of its cells, and find that we are incapable of understanding it. In this matter Kant's conviction will always remain true: "The formation of celestial bodies, the causes of their movements, and in short, the origin of the entire Cosmos, will be explained sooner than the mechanism of the creation of a plant or a caterpillar." The data which chemistry offers will likewise never lead us any further. Every man has in himself his own individual biological laws, every man bears with him his own psychological complexes. Consequently there are no psychological constants common to all individuals. The attempt to establish any such is foredoomed to failure. Thus it is impossible to foretell *a priori* the reaction between an organism and a given chemical body. It is significant that such a man as Kant realized the extreme importance of individual differences when writing to the physician, Marcus Herz: "Be sure to study the great diversity of human nature."

Tolerance and Habituation

The foregoing problem must be based on the same level as that of habit and custom, which has occupied philosophers since the earliest days of medicine. Habit includes somatic reactions which up to present day have not been satisfactorily explained. The point in question is that an agent capable of effecting a functional reaction in a certain portion of an animal organism under conditions constant in form and quality, has the intensity of its action reduced even to the point of inertia if its application be repeated.

This phenomena can be studied throughout organic life. If, by pressure on a part of the skin during rowing, for instance, pain and local irritation are produced, it can be ascertained that by repeating the irritating action the symptoms gradually decrease until an equal amount of mechanical influence is hardly felt. This may be, though it is not necessarily, the result of the callosities that are formed. It may be that the sensitive nerves react to a lesser degree to repeated influence of this kind even when not protected by a callosity. I have often seen gardeners in charge of cacti handle mamillaries or echinocacti without being inconvenienced by the many needles that pierced their hands, when an inexperienced person was forced to pull out even a single needle because of its irritation. There are many opportunities for studying similar functions of the sensitive nerves, especially in industry. Those whose work exposes them to the din of heavy machinery or the noise of looms experience no disagreeable sensations therefrom; similarly, soldiers in war become accustomed to the firing of guns and the detonation of exploding shells.

All sensitive organs subjected to the assault of a factor which uniformly irritates, excites, or effects a functional reaction in a certain degree, can, as is generally known, attain and manifest a dulling of susceptibility. The final result, i.e. the decrease of subjective sensitiveness, does not depend on the nature of the repeated active agent. It can be effected by any one of countless irritants. If we consider skin irritants, which apparently exercise the same influence on the same surface, we must admit that each acts differently from the other. Mechanical, luminous, thermal, and chemical action resemble each other in their final effect of establishing a habit or custom. The truth of this assertion may be ascertained by a short stay in the stokehole of a steamer. On the first occasion the heat radiated produces such a feeling of suffocation that an immediate exit is necessary, but if the experiment is repeated, the intolerable sensations disappear and even a lengthy stay imparts no ill-effects. After remaining in an accumulator-charging room for the first time it seems impossible for the mechanics to endure the foggy sulfurous vapors for any long period, because of their extremely irritating effect on the respiratory organs. Nevertheless, men who work there give no indication of inflammation of the mucous membranes produced by these fumes.

We might cite hundreds of examples of this kind, due to material influences, especially of a chemical nature. They find their analogy in other effects, verified by experience, due to psychological influences. In this field impressions differ in nature and intensity: e.g. disgust, fear, sorrow, and perhaps even love are diminished if their duration is prolonged. Psychological impressions ranging from extreme joy to extreme sorrow, from a state of good humor to a morbid disposition, lose their influence on the individual if they are active for any length of time. A habit is established, and the subjective manifestation of the senses, the response to the influence exercised, slowly disappears: "L'habitude émouse le sentiment."

But how, by what means and to what extent a habit may be established can never be absolutely determined. It must be considered as a law that the state of custom or habit ceases to remain constant when the intensity of the instigating agent is suddenly augmented. This is what occurs if, for instance, the magnitude or the aspect of a danger to which a person has become so accustomed that he neglects his power of judgment is unexpectedly changed, or if an acute increase of pain eliminates the former habitual insensibility. Habitual toleration therefore only exists in a limited amount and for a definite quantity of a habit-producing agent. That is why a sudden increase of that last innocuous dose of morphia, cocaine, nicotine, or caffeine, poisons the habitual drug-taker as much as if his organism had not acquired a relative immunity to the effect of these noxious substances by preceding prolonged use.

The influence of habit may be traced even in unicellular organisms. A freshwater amoebae dies if 2 per cent of salt is suddenly added to the water in which it lives. But if a progressive increase of 0.1 per cent of salt is added to the daily dose, the amoeba accustoms itself to the increasing concentration, and eventually is able to live in a 2 per cent solution. If it is returned to fresh water it dies. Sea-water amoebas and rhizopods continue to live even if the water, through vaporization in an open dish, reaches a 10 per cent concentration of salt. The growth of yeast in beer is arrested by 0.17 gr. of hydrofluoric acid per litre, whereas when accustomed to this substance it can tolerate 1 gr. per litre. The bacillus of pneumonia is destroyed by a sublimate solution of 1 in 15,000, but after accommodation thereto will continue its development in a solution of 1 in 2,000.

The plasmodia of *aethalium septicum* can be accustomed to solutions of sugar. The fungus *aspergillus niger* accommodates itself to a nutrient medium with an increasing salt content, and, by slowly increasing the concentration, to a solution containing 28 per cent sodium nitrate and even 52 per cent glycerol. After a prolonged development in contact with nickel sulfate, another fungus, *penicillium glaucum*, tolerates ten times the quantity which would at the beginning prevent its growth. It can likewise be accustomed to cobalt, cadmium, mercury, and thallium salts. Fungi can likewise be accustomed to concentrations of 2 to 8 per cent ethyl alcohol, or even amylic or other noxious alcohols, by suitably regulating and increasing the quantity which at the beginning is toxic. While 0.1 per cent amylic alcohol prevents all fructification, *penicillium* accustomed to it continues to fructify in a nutritive medium containing 0.4 per cent of this substance. In a solution of 0.005 per cent morphia, *rhizopus nigricans* grows well. Higher concentrations hinder its development. However, after being prepared for only five days, it will thrive in a solution containing 0.5 per cent. The plasmodia of *physarum* establish a habit in respect of arsenious acid, which is at first detrimental, and *penicillium brevicaule* and some other fungi have the property, so important in juridicial chemistry, of transforming this noxious acid into gaseous odoriferous products.

Higher organisms also manifest a certain tolerance of different poisons established through habit or custom. Rabbits can become accustomed to jerquirity seeds (abrin) to such an extent as to endure without any general disturbance of the body an infusion of four times the quantity that would normally cause death. Dogs and rabbits can even be habituated to a certain extent to curare by slowly increasing the dose. It is necessary to augment rapidly the quantity administered in order to evoke the toxic symptoms which appeared after the first doses. Horses at first strongly affected by the presence of *galeopsis tetrahit* in their fodder become fully accustomed to it.

A large number of similar examples might be cited; for instance, corresponding results have been observed in animals which have been treated with atropine, the active principle of *atropa belladonna*. If dogs are subjected for a longer period of time to the toxic action of greater or lesser quantities of this substance, it may be observed after a few days that a series of general symptoms, e.g. hyperaesthesia of the skin, trembling of the whole body, restlessness, etc., have disappeared. After 5 to 10 injections of atropine they cannot be distinguished from completely normal, unpoisoned animals. Even a substance like dimethyl sulphate, with its violently caustic action, may be given to rabbits which have been slowly inured to it, in doses of 0˙15 or 0˙2 gr. per day, without causing rapid intoxication, whereas 0˙075 gr. is sufficient to kill others within twenty-four hours.

Animals exposed to the action of carbon monoxide gas for the first time manifested greater sensibility than those accustomed to it, e.g. as regards the temperature of the body.

In the same way, a habit can be established in respect of physical factors, such as the rarefied air on the summit of mountains. In certain places in Bolivia, Bogotà, Potosì, La Paz, and others which are situated at an altitude of 2,600 to 4,000 metres, it can be ascertained that the inhabitants do not differ in physical fitness from the people of the plains. The heights in question are equal to that of Mont Blanc, where Saussure hardly had the strength to read his instruments, and his guides and experienced mountaineers fainted. Whereas the individual not inured to these heights exhibits during absolute repose, and to a greaater extent during exercise, an acceleration of the pulse accompanied by palpitation of the heart and general oppression, the accommodated pulse becomes normal after eight to ten days with only an increase of its tension. The respiration behaves in the same way: at first it is more frequent, later normal.

Such an adaptation to great altitudes took place to a most striking extent among those who tried to ascend Mount Everest in 1922. First breathing difficulties and headaches were experienced, and, at a height of 5,000 metres, Cheyne-Stokes respiration. Ten or so superficial respirations were succeeded by others which gradually became deeper and culminated in three or four deep breaths; these gradually decreased in depth until the series started again with superficial respirations. After a sojourn of some weeks all disagreeable sensations disappeared. The rate of accommodation is not interrupted by difficult or strenuous mountaineering. After a few days, adaptation takes place at a height of 6,400 metres, and the difficulties which at first seemed too great are overcome with ease; it becomes possible to reach 8,400 meters without using oxygen. Accommodation even at this altitude takes place very rapidly.

Another instance: in South Brittany the air is laden with salt to such an extent that some persons are attacked after a few days by a painful affection similar to colic. After three to eight days these symptoms vanish, never to appear again.

There is hardly a tissue in the whole body which, by suitable treatment, cannot be made to tolerate an otherwise noxious substance, and hardly an agent capable of altering the functions of an organism which cannot by habitual administration lose in whole or in part its influence on the tissues in question. According to my experience, those substances which destroy the structure of haemoglobin and phosphorous seem to be the only exceptions.

But, as I have already stated, this accommodation of the tissue takes place only to a certain degree or in the case of certain substances, whereas it may be completely absent of other substances whose action is similar. Nevertheless, this experimental law has many exceptions. Oil of croton, rubbed into the skin of the ear of a rabbit, for some weeks causes a kind of immunity which manifests itself by a lesser degree of response to the same kind of irritation after the primary inflammation has disappeared. It could be proved that a preparatory treatment with other substances producing inflammation provided a greater resistance against the action of the oil of croton, and that conversely a preliminary inflammation caused by oil of croton offered a certain degree of protection against other irritants of the skin. This habit of immunity with regard to these substances can be formed without any apparent inflammation, and continues for some weeks. It does not, however, disappear after the same length of time in respect of all agents capable of evoking a cutaneous inflammation, but endures longest for that substance to which the animal had been systematically accustomed. Analogous results were obtained by experimenting on man. If psoriasis is treated with the irritant chrysarobin in slowly increased concentrations, the portions of skin concerned become less sensitive not only to chrysarobin but also to other irritants, e.g. oil of croton and cantharides plaster. It was ascertained that the tolerance of one patient for the latter substances had disappeared, whereas it remained for weeks in the case of chrysarobin. Laboratory and clinical experiments lead to the same conclusions in this respect. They teach us that the organism in hundreds and thousands of different forms can be adapted by habit to the most diverse influences. This is true both with regard to isolated organs, e.g. the brain, and to the organism as a whole. It is known that the seeds of *strychnos ignatii* and *strychnos nux vomica,* which are rich in strychnine, have been taken regularly for years in the East as a prophylactic against snake-bite and cholera.

How can this phenomenon be explained? As a matter of course, the cause which produces the phenomenon of habit cannot at the same time be the reason of the habit itself; this must be sought for in the individual concerned. Nearly 400 years before the Christian era, we find it stated that "the effect of all medicinal and poisonous plants is diminished through habit. Sometimes they become quite ineffective. Human nature triumphs over them as if they were not poisons." The human body is here considered, by virtue of its organization, as capable of destroying the toxic powers of the drug. Some centuries later Galen expressed other views. He relates how an old woman of Athens grew used to hemlock by consuming small quantities, and later was able to take very large amounts with impunity, because "at the beginning the organism conquered the poison when taken in small doses, because of their minuteness, and habit afterwards made it a kindred, naturally assimilated substance."[2]

Many theories are possible with regard to the ultimate reason for the formation of a habit, for instance that of taking morphia or similar drugs. I reject those which assert the likelihood of an "anti-toxin" being formed in the blood-serum in proportion to the quantity of the drug habitually taken.

According to this hypothesis, the protecting substance is produced in such abundance that other persons can, if necessary make use of the antitoxic qualities of this serum with benefit to themselves. This supposition is all the more unreasonable because every cellular complex subjected to a chronic intoxication invariably succumbs to the poisoning in the end, in spite of an initial increase of resistance due to self-defense.

Indeed, a number of important experiments, my own among others, have proved that antitoxins are not formed against alkaloids, glycosides, substances of the aliphatic or aromatic series, or inorganic substances. Neither a cocaine- nor a morphia-antitoxin is produced in the blood, and if we are told that a so-called antitoxin serum has been prepared from animals chronically poisoned with one or other of these substances, we must suppose that scientific observation in this case was inadequate. No branch of science is more liable to insufficient experimental technique than that in question. The sad craze for conjecture is apt to spread like a contagious disease, and imitators, of whom the world is full, easily suggest themselves into finding what they want to find, because others before them believed that they had discovered the truth. If one of these antitoxic serums has really produced a temporary symptomatic success in a patient, we must attribute this to the heterogeneous albumen injected. This explanation, which I was the first to put forward,[3] has since been accepted by very many scientists. It also holds good in respect to "curative sera" which do not contain any specific antitoxin.

I likewise regard as unproven and fallacious the idea that the formation of a habit with regard to poisons like morphia can be attributed to the increasing ability to destroy the morphia which the organism acquires, and depends upon this ability. The following test is sufficient to refute this presumption. The brain of a rat, which had been immunized against morphia, contained, one hour after the administration of a dose which evoked no symptoms whatever, a greater quantity of the poison than that of a non-immunized animal which succumbed to the same dose.

I have repeatedly stated my opinion about the drug-habit and its nature,[4] and it has become public property to such an extent that many who have written on this problem at a later date, and recognized my statements as true, thought that they were expressing their own ideas. The following will illustrate my views.

If we suppose that a substance capable of provoking a reaction exercises its influence on certain cellular complexes of the organism, then an unusual functional reaction is produced which can more or less be identified. The return to the normal state takes place as soon as the tissues affected have come to rest, and as soon as the irritating influence has moreover been eliminated. But if the administration of a substance endowed with chemical energy is frequently repeated, neither of the above-indicated phenomena take place. Every new dose introduced into the organism still finds remains of the preceding doses and eventually a modified functional ability of the affected part.[5] Whereas a healthy cell, because of its life, i.e. through its physical or chemical elasticity, is enabled to triumph in a certain degree and for a certain time over non-assimilable foreign bodies and their effects, it becomes impossible, if the introduction of the substance is constantly repeated, for the perpetually incapacitated cell to return to a state of rest. Besides this, its normal functional ability to ward off the foreign body which exercises a hostile paralyzing or irritating influence is slowly but surely diminished. Every new dose acts on a basis whose capacity for functional reaction is reduced. In order to maintain this reaction at the required level, it is necessary to increase the dose progressively, and thus the energy of the cell is numbed over and over again until, after this process has lasted a certain time and a fixed quantity of the substance, varying with the individual, has been absorbed, the vital powers of the cell permit only of vegetation, i.e. allow it to live but do not suffice to ensure its protection against the incessant noxious influence or its normal physiological activity, which includes the necessary intimate relationship with other organs of the body.

According to my interpretation, therefore, the drug-habit, which I regard as a purely vital function, is not based upon an increase in energy of the cells, but, on the contrary, on a weakening of cellular vitality caused probably by chemical influences. Adaptation is the acquired incapacity to respond in a normal manner to a specific degree of excitation.

This weakness of the disarmed cell, the result of progressive adaptation, produces a certain degree of immunity from the toxic action of the irritating agent. If, by excessive administration of the poison, the limit of tolerance is surpassed, the toxic effects appear as with non-adapted persons.

The vegetative functions of the defective group of cells are threatened in their existence, and disturbances of the functions of other cells, which are subject to their regulating influence, can be ascertained. There exists in a healthy state, on the other hand, harmonious co-operation between the functions of the organs of the body.

This organic relationship may be compared with a limited company, in which the single shareholders have a greater or lesser influence, but nevertheless all work together with one object in view: the conversation of the normal vital functions of the body. If one of the partners comes to grief, the others are also involved, and do their utmost to compensate for the initial damage up to the limit of their capability. Eventually they are exhausted, and each one takes the luckless path which destiny has assigned him. The bond which connected them is severed, and it will be difficult if not impossible to unite the company again. These diseases, due to the interdependence of the tissues, may result from any morbid disorder, and become worse than the primary affection.

If the functions of the brain, for example, have been brought through habit to a modified state, then every decrease in the quantity of the drug to which the habit has accustomed it disturbs the artificially established equilibrium with regard to the toleration of the foreign influence. The life of the cell has adapted itself to or was dominated by the drug, and if it is lacking a craving appears.

This reminds us of the hunger for salt which may be observed when a person has been deprived of this substance for some time. Just as the body needs to be supplied with this substance, which is an indispensable component of it, so certain narcotic or other substances become through their habitual employment integral substances of the brain, and the lack of them is felt in the same way as that of a necessary ingredient of the body. Thus we may say that morphia becomes a "hormone" for a morphinist. It enters into the community of the body, and is, as Galen said, σύμφυτον. For instance, a certain person was able during a period of three years to pour 0.1 to 0.2 gr. of quinine four to six times a day on his tongue and swallow it without water. When asked the reason of this strange habit, he replied that he liked the effect of the substance. If he ceased to take it he became flurried and could not fulfill his professional duties. The same was probably the case with that old woman of whom Galen states that she gradually habituated herself to "cicuta" (i.e. presumably spotted cowbane and not water hemlock). In the same manner the people whom the Spaniards encountered on the coast of Peru made use of caustic lime in order to stimulate the organs of taste. The Goajiros at the mouth of the Rio la Hacha, and others, do the same at the present day. A deprivation of this irritant causes internal disorders of a general nature.

We can but put forward bare hypotheses as to whether the action of these substances depends upon their absorption in the cells[6] or whether any alternative explanation may be supposed. I do not see the necessity for such a supposition, especially since signs of the chemical affinity of the substances in question, morphia, cocaine, etc., to cellular bodies have been sought for in vain. But even if this were otherwise, it would in no respect alter my analytical interpretation of the process, for it is really immaterial to the final result whether there takes place a combination with the cell or simply an exertion of energy by contact. It is essential only that the cell be brought under the influence of one of these substances.

The influence is removed by suppressing the drug in question. Then in the most favorable case the cell, thanks to the energies with which it is still provided or which it receives anew from life, can recover its former functional integrity, in the same way as a person, after being anæsthetized with ether or chloroform, comes back to a normal state when the anesthetic has been eliminated, although the functional activity of the ganglion-cells of his brain was temporarily diminished or suspended. Nevertheless, a certain modification of the functional constitution of the cell may have been established which does not disappear, and which may, when occasion arises, reveal itself by an easy relapse into the former state of dependence on the toxic agent. The reason for the relapse in such individuals is generally the remembrance of the agreeable sensations experienced when making use of the substance. The will-power, in the cellular life similar to that which so vividly preserves the agreeable impressions, cannot resist the attraction of a fresh dose of the drug, and a relapse occurs.

These material influences resemble in large measure those which we find in the spiritual life. Love of a woman, for instance, may degenerate into a passion for which there is no justification and which changes the life of the lover in regard of his judgment, will-power, and activity to such an extent that even the restraints of nature are thrust aside. Adaptation to this altered emotional life, even if it is inconvenient for the individual, is certain to take place with greater rapidity the more frequently the personal impression of the beloved object makes itself felt. If the woman who occasioned this state can be completely removed from the lover's horizon, an irritable weakness remains which prevents the rapid recovery of his normal faculties. He lives in the remembrance of the past, and though this may fade, the old passion with all its consequences is re-kindled as soon as the woman he loves appears again before his eyes.

The narcotic substances differ greatly among themselves with regard to the agreeable sensations they produce as inducements for their habitual use. These differences account for the degree of craving which they excite, but it has been found impossible to give an explanation of this. Such an explanation can probably be found in very delicate dissimilarities in the exciting qualities. So far we have discovered as the cause of the action of these substances and the resulting habitual adaptation, only functional reactions of the cell, which we must interpret in the last resort as chemical reactions. Morphological changes in the cell have so far not been demonstrated. All these cases in which so-called modifications in the microscopical structure of the cerebral or spinal tissues have been shown to occur are in my opinion based on errors in scientific judgment. Even in cases, for example, of adaptation to skin irritants, where the histology of the affected parts has been experimentally studied, no pathological modifications could be found. The narcotics do not leave any observable traces of their action in the nervous system. Nevertheless it is possible that modifications take place.

Immunity against Poisons

To the rich and varied field of personality in its widest sense appertain manifestations of immunity which, being innate, sometimes provide an apparently absolute protection against toxic or other factors. This immunity can, as described in the preceding pages, be realized, up to a certain limit if at all, through the formation of a habit by slowly increased dosage. It would even seem that this immunity is not merely peculiar to certain animal species, but that an analogous state can be produced in mankind. For instance, during long and dangerous epidemics it has been noticed that persons remain uninfected who must necessarily have absorbed some of the contagious matter. So far I am not certain of the existence of an immunity which *a priori* protects man against known noxious substances of a chemical nature. In all cases where an immunity of this kind has been thought to have been found, against the action of a toxic vapor, for example, there were probably certain external influences which prevented apparent toxic effects; or, on the other hand, the individuals concerned were hyposensitive and the quantity of the toxic agent insufficient. The very marked hyposensibility which can be ascertained towards, e.g. ethyl bromide, ethyl chloride, or chloroform should not be placed on the same level with the immunity we observe among certain animals to poisons which are capable of acting under all circumstances on man. In this respect the animal organism must be provided with certain peculiar quantities which allow for the absorption of proved poisons without apparent harm.

The hedgehog has long been considered as an animal extremely resistant to poisons. In fact, I have been able to prove[7] that although it can endure large quantities of cantharides or the venom of the common viper, this resistance is only relative. The viper itself seemed to be, during my experiments, not absolutely immune from its own venom; it could tolerate only certain quantities, and under these circumstances a retardation of the effect took place.

Nevertheless, there exist a considerable number of other observations which tend to confirm an absolute immunity towards certain poisons in the case of certain animals. If these are accurate, we cannot but suppose that the parts wherein the toxic action should be effective are differently conditioned from those of man or of other animals in which toxic reactions appear. The fungus *mucor rhizopodiformis*, for instance, poisons rabbits but has no effect on dogs. *Tylenchus tritici* thrives in glycerol, and belladonna, morphia, atropine, and strychnine do it no harm; on the other hand the salts of metals, acids, and alkalis have a detrimental effect. Ducks, hens, and doves are not poisoned by the internal application of opium. The rhinoceros-bird consumes the seeds of *stychnos nux vomica*, mice those of the bearded darnel, the blackbird belladonna, titmice the seeds of stramony, starlings those of spotted cowbane, rabbits and guinea-pigs the leaves and the fruit of belladonna.[8] Cows, sheep, and pigs, it is said, eat hembane, and snails the leaves of belladonna. The larva of *deïopeïa pulchella* derives its nourishment from the highly poisonous calabar bean. The caterpillars of *ornithoptera darsius* consume a poisonous aristolochia from which the poison is supposed to be transformed to the butterfly. The oleandor caterpillar eats the poisonous leaves of the plant from which it is named, and *cimex hyoscyami* the leaves of henbane. It is said that wild boars devour fern-roots, that rabbits are refractory to hashish, and that in Guadeloupe horses ravenously consume the leaves of *rhus toxicodendron*, which cause severe inflammation in man. In the Caucasus goats and sheep eat veratrum or hellebore, which intoxicates cows and horses.

The reaction of certain animals to low temperatures must also be placed among these enigmas. The "glacier flea," *desoria glacialis*, can not only jump about on the snowfields but remains in a frozen state for weeks and months at a temperature of −11°C without losing any of its vital energy. The snow flea of the plains, *degeeria*, can do the same. And they are composed of albumen! On the other hand, the common flea is unable to endure the climate of Tierra del Fuego, and perishes on being imported—a pleasant reflection for the ladies of the island!

Everywhere in this sphere of the difference in or absence of reaction of living matter to foreign or indigenous influences we are confronted with insoluble riddles. It is impossible to find the answer to them but it is necessary to become acquainted with the infinitely diverse forms in which they present themselves. Those which are connected with the narcotic and stimulating drugs should be of interest to everyone, even to those who exhibit selfish indifference. They constitute one of the world's problems, and those who are concerned in its solution—as who is not ?—must of necessity co-operate, consciously or otherwise.

NARCOTIC SUBSTANCES

Mode of Action

The substances whose effects I have in a general manner just described may be divided into several groups which, though not absolutely distinct, exhibit differences in the nature and manifestations of their energy. It will easily be understood that if an influence is exercised on the brain, its different parts may react differently although the effective agents seem to produce the same result. Even if we confess that the identity of the effects is not real, but that owing to the unsatisfactory means of investigation there is an apparent identity, there still remain enough experimentally proved toxicological facts to indicate that the chemical constitution of the various parts of the brain cannot be considered as identical. There must be quantitative and qualitative chemical differences in both the gray and the white matter of the brain. Chemical investigations up to the present have told us very little as to this. They inform us that the quantity of neuralgia and albumen represents more than half the organic matter of the gray substance and only a quarter of that of the white substance, that the quantity of cholesterol and fatty matter is only one-third of the gray substance, and that the proportion of cerebrin, approximately one-twentieth, is the same as in the white substance, etc. Even if the substances mentioned were really integral constituents of the cerebral tissues and not the result of chemical analysis, then we are enlightened only as to the chemical constitution of the dead brain and not in the least as to the function on which the activity of the brain is based. If, as I think, there are differences, it can be understood why substances which exert an influence on the brain evoke diverse effects in quality and quantity in its different departments. Cholesterol, phoshatide, cephaline, cerebroside are only names which we apply to substances whose active part in the functional process of the normal or morbid brain we cannot understand.

Several toxic processes have brought me to the conclusion that there are differences also in the vital requirements of the various parts of the brain. It has been impossible to understand, even approximately, why in the case of carbon monoxide poisoning it is the ganglions of the base which are most affected, especially the corpus striatum and also the thalamus and copora quadrigemina. The simplest explanation would be to suppose that these parts of the brain have a greater need of blood that is rich in oxygen and undeteriorated, and cannot be satisfied with blood containing carbon monoxide. At the same time perhaps we may assume an increased chemical reactivity towards substances which are produced by disintegration of the aforementioned parts through malnutrition.

The functional response of the spinal bulb, for instance, towards narcotics, is an example of the differences which can be ascertained with regard to the reactive capacity towards certain chemical substances of single parts or points of the brain. Whereas the centres of the cerebral cortex react by a rapid cessation of certain of their functions, more time and a greater mass of the effective agent is necessary in order to bring about a functional modification of the respiratory centre. These various results should not be attributed solely to the size of the dose administered, for if the law of mass action can undoubtedly be applied to a certain extent to the medicinal and toxic action of drugs, its importance cannot be compared with the part it plays in chemistry.

A primary excitation should be included among the constant reactions of the brain to narcotics. I regard it as a general law of biology that a diminution of the functions of any organ of the body is preceded by an increase of functional energy, the expression of the primary excitation. The force and duration of this excitation depends upon the state of the individual brain and the nature of the exciting agent. It is always there, even if it cannot by ordinary means be perceived, and may be so considerable as to represent for some time the only determinable reaction.

Besides the direct effects on the central nervous system brought about by the substances in question, there are, as I have already stated, effects which extend to the other organic functions, and may be called secondary effects.

If we consider the great and permanent influence exercised by the brain and spinal cord on the life of the organism, on the heart and respiration, the glands, the muscles, the sense-organs, etc., and if it is true, as I believe, that even the processes of nutrition and assimilation are dependent on the nervous centres, it will be evident without further explanation that the action of narcotic substances will also be felt in the organs which are under the influence of the nervous system. The symptoms which result from this dependence, combined with the manifestations of direct action on the brain and spinal cord, form the clinical record of the effects of these substances.

The final explanation of the mode of action on the brain is far from having as yet been found. It has even been found impossible to theorize on the phenomena of artificial sleep or the anæsthesia of pain. None of the numerous attempts at explanation deserve to be quoted. They are nothing else than the circumscription of the process itself and merely provoke ridicule. Is it a chemical process which takes place in the nervous substance of the cerebral cortex? This is my view, although it is urged against this opinion that the minute quantities of the active substance introduced into the organism which bring about such evident effects would not be sufficient to cause a chemical reaction to take place. I regard this objection as not having sufficient support to refute my point of view. For even if half a milligramme of scopolamine is a very small quantity compared with the mass of the brain to bring about a cerebral action in the form of somnolence, we must not forget the action probably affects certain definite centres which are no more than points in the brain. The narcotic may have on these limited points a catalytic action, i.e. without producing any chemical change it may cause paralysis or excitation so long as it remains in contact with the centre capable of being influenced. We may easily conclude that scopolamine or morphia may arrest or accelerate normal functions which would, in this case, lead to sleep.

The chemical action of one group of these substances, the anesthetics that are inhaled, is more accessible, because they possess the recognizable property of dissolving the fatty matter of the brain, a property which can be regarded as also capable of promoting a functional modification. This explanation of the mode of action of these substances, which I gave many years ago,[1] and which has been adopted by others and put forward as their own, has a high degree of probability. The rapidity of the re-establishment of the normal state after the cessation of the toxic action, which remains unexplained, cannot be understood. But if we admit that a catalytic action by contact exists, as is possible with other substances of the same group, there will be no difficulty in understanding the re-establishment of the normal state.

Classifications of
Narcotic and Stimulating Drugs

I classify the agents capable of effecting a modification of the cerebral functions, and used to obtain at will agreeable sensations of excitement or peace of mind, as follows:

First group: Euphorica; sedatives of mental activity. These substances diminish or even suspend the functions of emotion and perception in their widest sense, sometimes reducing or suppressing, sometimes conserving consciousness, inducing in the person concerned a state of physical and mental comfort. To this group belong opium and its components, morphia, codeine, etc., and cocaine.

Second group: Phantastica; hallucinating substances. This series comprises a number of substances of vegetable origin, varying greatly in their chemical constitution, and to these belongs in its proper sense the name Phantastica, or Drugs of Illusion. The representatives of this group, such as mescal buttons *(anhalonium lewinii),* Indian hemp *(cannabis indica),* and the plants which contain tropines, bring about evident cerebral excitation in the form of hallucinations, illusions, and visions. These phenomena may be accompanied or followed by unconsciousness or other symptoms of altered cerebral functioning.

Third group: Inebriantia. These bodies can be produced by chemical synthesis (e.g. alcohol, chloroform, ether, benzine). A primary phase of cerebral excitation is followed by a state of depression which may eventually extend to complete temporary suppression of the functions.

Fourth group: Hyponitca; sleep-producing agents, such as chloral, veronal, sulphonal, etc.

Fifth group: Excitantia; mental stimulants. Substances of vegetable origin which produce without alteration of consciousness a generally more or less apparent excitation of the brain. To this series belong the plants containing caffeine, tobacco, betel, etc.

EUPHORICA: MENTAL SEDATIVES

Opium: Morphia

Opium and Morphia as Euphorics: Their History, Production, and Effect

The use of opium and its ingredients as a soothing and euphoric remedy has developed into a grave menace to the life of nations. Differing from alcoholism in that it does not betray its victim to others, the opium habit, especially since the war, has taken hold of whole classes of people who were formerly free from it. This abuse has almost become epidemic, and has moved from various States, in their capacity as guardians of the public health, to take measures of defence against it. Germany is no better than any other country in this respect, for there is nothing which man can do for good or ill which is not common to all nations.

The discussion of these problems necessitates a wider knowledge than the man in the street possesses. The contents of the following pages are derived from my personal researches in narcotics and other drugs of the same kind, and my observations of many persons who had become slaves to this passion both on the coasts of the Pacific and in Europe.

By this passion I mean the state which induces persons, habitually and as the result of a violent craving, to employ opium, morphia, and other substances of the same kind, without being driven thereto by a grave or incurable disease, but with the sole object of obtaining agreeable sensations in the brain, even though they know, or ought to know, that they are risking health and life as the price of this abuse.

This definition distinguishes between those who make use of the drug because of chronic incurable disease, and the morpinist in the usual sense of the word, a sense bearing a certain reproach; but it includes those who become ill through their use of the drug.

In contradistinction from the morally degenerative passsions, such as gambling, the passion for drugs has an actual material basis—namely, the substance in question, which affects the functions of the brain. Of all the consequences which may be inferred, one is decisive: the loss of the will to resist the attraction of morphia, cocaine, etc. The effects which these substances call forth are so agreeable that moral resistance is overcome. The question whether morphia and similar drugs, by momentarily reinforcing the activity of the brain, enable the individual to meet more satisfactorily the increasing demands of the world of to-day and to succeed in the struggle for existence, must be answered in the negative. The substances which temporarily produce these effects are of another species; they are excitants which act on the brain in another way.

Opium and morphia occupy a singular and unparalleled position among medicinal substances, and the little we know of their history, very incomplete as it is, is no less extraordinary. The documents that would supply these gaps are lacking, but our present knowledge of the pharmacology and toxicology of these substances furnishes us with inductive elements of relationship and enables us to reconstruct their history completely.

Relics from the obscure period of the Stone Age, the epoch of the lake-dwellers of some 4,000 years ago, are from time to time discovered. For instance, in the Swiss lakes not only seeds but also capsules of poppies have been found. The examination of these capsules suggests the conclusion that they came not from the primitive form of the poppy, *papaver setigerum*, but were obtained by cultivation. It is impossible to decide whether the cultivation was brought about in order to obtain the oil of the seeds or merely the narcotic juice of the capsules. But the second alternative is to be considered. We cannot reject it, since a knowledge of the narcotic effect of the juice of the poppy might easily be acquired while cultivating the plant, for instance as a result of tasting from curiousity the juice flowing from an accidental incision in the capsule. The further step to its use as an anodyne is not a very long one. But in that case the inhabitants of the

Swiss lakes would indeed occupy a singular position among the lake-dwellers.

Sounder and more conclusive material for the study of the knowledge and use of opium in antiquity may be found in very ancient documents, for instance in Homer. In his time the use of nepenthes, the drug of forgetfulness, was already so well known that the first discovery of the effects of opium must probably be dated back to a very much earlier age. For nepenthes was a preparation of opium, although other interpretations have been given by persons unacquainted with the decisive effects of opium, among others by philologists.

It is stated in the *Odyssey* that when Telemachus visited Menelaus in Sparta, the remembrance of Ulysses and other warriors acted very depressingly on the assembly. Menelaus then ordered a banquet to be served, and Helen prepared a peculiar drink.

> And Helen, daughter of Zeus, poured into the wine they were drinking a drug, nepenthes, which gave forgetfulness of evil. Those who had drunk of this mixture did not shed a tear the whole day long, even though their mother or father were dead, even though a brother or a beloved son had been killed before their eyes by weapons of the enemy. And the daughter of Zeus possessed this wonderful substance which Polydamna had given to her, the wife of Thos in Egypt, that fertile country which produced so many balms, some beneficial and some deadly.

There is only one substance in the world capable of acting this way, and that is opium, the vehicle of morphia. Its characteristic effect, especially after habitual use, is precisely such a state of indifference towards everything except the ego. The execellent description of this state which Homer gives is apparently the result of observing opium-eaters, i.e. people who habitually use opium for their pleasure. For the first dose as a rule does not produce these effects on the emotional life, and even if produced, they would not be of such long duration. It is not poetic licence, but observation from real life, when the poet says that those who were under the permanent influence of opium were free from emotions of the soul the whole day.

The description enables us to make another assumption, that warriors consumed nepenthes before battle in order to dull their senses of danger, for Homer here speaks only of the numbing of the soul towards the horrors of combat. This might have happened, and in my opinion did happen, before Troy and elsewhere. A connection is thus established with the employment of opium for the same purpose hundreds and thousands of years later. Only the initiated, the "heroes," made use of it. Indeed, this substance and the knowledge of its action was not accessible to everybody. Surely Helen had prepared this opiate at other times and on other occasions for her confidants. It was the Egyptian Polydamna who procured it and from whom she learnt its use. This is an important indication of the country which first produced poppies.[1]

In the papyrus of Ebers we find a chapter with the title "Remedy to prevent the excessive crying of children." It will be seen that for this purpose špenn is used: "špenn, the grains of the špenn plant, with the excretions of flies found on the wall, strained to a pulp, passed through a sieve and administered on four successive days. The crying will stop at once." The theory that the action is based on opium is well founded. Either the unripe seeds—the ripe ones are useless—or the capsule of the poppy were employed. To-day, both in Egypt and Europe, children are still "soothed" with the aid of this product, and not infrequently the effects are fatal.

The cultivation of opium, then, probably spread over Asia Minor, which land is called to-day, though without proof, the cradle of opium. From there the poppy reached Rome, Greece, and other parts. In Egypt, as in India, the right of prescribing and supplying opium must have been in primitive times, as a piece of occult knowledge, a privilege of the priests. Many obscure events of history can be unraveled by the light we receive from the fact that the action of opium was known. At the beginning these very powerful medicines were used for philanthropic purposes, and later they often served political or personal ends and the designs of passion and vengeance.[2] Representations of poppies were often engraved on Roman coins of the later ages. In Jewish history they have only been found on the bronze coins of John Hyrcanus, prince and high-priest of the race of the Maccabees (135–106 B.C.)

The seductive power of opium, which incites an incessant renewal of its use, as millions of experiences and human nature itself prove, found its victims in Rome and in Greece, who desired a state of mental detachment from the life of the world. The short descriptions which are given to us by the naturalists Theophrastus (third century B.C.), Pliny, and Dioscorides (first century A.D.) show that the toxic effects of the drug which were judged so important that Diagoras of Melos and Erasistratus, in the fifth and third centuries before Christ, recommended the complete avoidance of its use. But the employment of

Lethaeo perfusa papavera somno [3]

"poppies soaked with sleep of Lethe," has never been abandoned. Not only the dragon which dwelt in and protected the garden of the Hesperides, lying in the far-off country of the Moors, where the sunsets and the huge mountain Atlas bears the heavens on his shoulders, succumbed to its action:

Spargens humida melle soporiferumque papaver [4]

. . . "gave him inebriating poppy with dewy honey," but also innumerable human beings.

It is interesting to note that the poppy-head belonged to the mysteries of Ceres, for she took papaver "to forget the pain," *ad oblivionem doloris.* That is why a small earthen statue of Ceres-Isis with a torch holds poppy-heads in her hand.[5] Everywhere in antique art we meet with the poppy as a mythological symbol of sleep, and even a personification of the dispenser of sleep, the god who gives sleep, the ὑπνοδότης; he is presented as a bearded man leaning over the sleeper and pouring on his eyelids the poppy-juice contained in a vessel of horn which he holds in his hand.

On the coffin of the sleeping Ariadne, the bearded God of Sleep is holding poppy-heads and an opium-horn in his hand. At a later date the God of Sleep, Somnus, is depicted as a young genie carrying poppies and an opium-horn, or with a poppy-stalk in his hand.

In order to keep Hannibal away from Rome and to overpower him with dreams, Juno cries:

Per tenebras portas medicata papavera cornu . . . quatit inde soporas
Devexo capiti pennas, oculisque quietem
Irrorat tangens Lethaea tempora virga. [6]

Night and Sleep live both in the same dwelling, which, according to Lucian's romantic picture, is surrounded by a plantation of poppies. They appear with the sinking sun with a wreath of poppies round their heads, followed by a flock of dreams, and pour on man the soporific poppy-juice which binds his limbs.

The eating of opium, which has been practised here and there ever since the discovery of its effects, increased in proportion to the wider knowledge of the beneficial properties of the substance. How could it be otherwise? Ceasing to be the exclusive property of a minority, it lost its mystery and became a common object of commerce. It exercised its attraction of necessity, leading people to a first trial and consequently to the first step towards the habit. Time has preserved some testimonies of this abuse, which in all periods has shunned the light. It is stated, for example, in the second century, that Lysis took four drachms of poppy-juice without being incommoded.[7] He must have been an inveterate opium-eater; such toleration would otherwise have been impossible. In a period of the great Arabic doctors of the tenth–thirteenth centuries, and in consequence of the warlike expeditions of the Mohammedans, the passion for opium was propagated from Asia Minor to almost every part of the world. The considerable successes of Paracelsus, the miraculous cures which he effected with the aid of opium at the beginning of the sixteenth century, no doubt produced many opium-eaters; perhaps even Paracelsus himself took opium. "I posses a secret remedy which I call laudanum and which is superior to all other heroic remedies." His later life and way of acting create the impression of an opium-eater. I think it is very near the truth; I have seen many morphinists whose behaviour was similar.

In the year 1546, a French naturalist, Belon, who had travelled through Asia Minor and Egypt, drew attention to the great development of the abuse of opium among the Turks. "There is no Turk who would not buy opium with his last penny; he carries it on him in war and in peace. They eat opium because they think that they thus become more daring and have less fear of the dangers of war. In war-time such quantities are purchased that it is difficult to find any left." Belon saw an opium-eater take 2 gr. in one dose, and when he gave him 4 gr., accurately weighed, he consumed these at once without inconvenience. At this period opium was already exported on a large scale to Persia, India, and Europe. Belon reports that at that time fifty camels laden with opium proceeded to the two former regions. Whatever the motive for its use, the Portuguese botanist Garcias ab Horto, at the beginning of the sixteenth century, mentions the suppression of disagreeable physical and mental impressions experienced by the Indian opium-eaters whose acquaintance he made at Goa, and he even observed that when they had taken a sufficient quantity "They spoke wisely about all sorts of things. Such is the power of habit."

The importation of this substance into Europe from the East increased the numbers of those who used it, and, while probably taken in the first place as a medicine, it never ceased to hold its victims captive. I have found publications from the sixteenth–eighteenth centuries according to which persons had been medically observed in Germany who were "addicted to opium-eating" and consumed up to 40 gr. a day, and only showed signs of "lassitude and sleepiness." Some of these are reported to have continued the consumption of opium in increasing doses for a number of years, one woman, for example, taking in forty years 63 pounds of "fluid opium," i.e. tincture of opium. Another consumed 4 gr. a day for nineteen years, 27 kilos in all. A third, led to use it as an anodyne by an accident, is said to have introduced 100 kilos of the drug into his system in the course of thirty-four years.

Prosper Alphini at the end of the sixteenth century reports that some Egyptians consumed 12 gr. of opium a day without inconvenience.[8] Later, in the seventeenth century, for instance, medical men such as Sydenham enthusiastically propagated opium by recommendation and this not only against painful diseases. Eventually opium was considered as the "Hand of God," or the "Sacred anchor of life."

Save for some medical reports, we have only a few personal observations originating from the multitude who in the following centuries became slaves to opium and succumbed to it. One of these is by an English writer, De Quincey.[9] At the age of seventeen he began taking tincture of opium against neuralgic pains. For eight years he experienced no harm, and then entered a stage where the "Divine Poppy-juice became as indispensable as breathing," and took a glassful every day mixed with port wine and water. Renewed physical suffering made him "a confirmed opium-eater." After another eight years he daily consumed 8,000 drops, about 20 gr., of the tincture. In one of the following years which was "a year of brilliant water set and insulated in the gloomy umbrage of opium" he managed to diminish the daily dose to one-eighth. This was for a long time the last glimpse of the light in his life, which he spent under this magic spell. In spite of a fresh increase in the doses administered, he thought he was indebted to opium for his times of happiness—until the miseries and tortures of opium began.

This misery all such must experience. They have sold themselves body and soul. The proceeds of the sale are rapidly squandered in the delights of opium. These delights are inexorably followed by a state of individual physical and mental torture, of remorse mingled with grief.

This the English poet Coleridge discovered, who on some days consumed 20 to 25 gr. of tincture of opium. The same lot befell Francis Thompson, one of the most gifted younger English poets.

It is well known also that some medical men have been addicted to opium. It was known even in those times that habitual opium-eaters could not be deceived when their opium was replaced by other substances because, like the morphinists of to-day, they thereby experienced "unbearable pains."

So early as the eighth century the Arabs brought opium and the knowledge of its effects, by way of Persia, to India and China—to China which represents numerically a quarter of the earth's population. Before the Tang dynasty it was unknown. In the year 973 it was officially mentioned in the medical book *K'ai-pao-pên-tsäo* under the name of *ying-tzü-su*, and at the same time we find a poppy beverage recommended in a poem of Su Tung-P'a which gives us the impression that it alludes to other and more agreeable effects than the cure of dysentery, etc. At the beginning of the twelfth century cakes of opium were prepared from the dried milky juice of the poppy in the form of a fish, certainly not for medicinal purposes alone. In the latter part of the fifteenth century there existed in China an important traffic in opium, both imported and home produced. Towards the end of the Ming dynasty—the last Ming emperor reigned from 1628 to 1644—when the smoking of tobacco was prohibited, the practice of smoking opium made its appearance. Later this was modified, as an ambassador sent to China in 1793 reports, and the habit of smoking tobacco mixed with a small amount of opium was established. When in 1729 two hundred chests of opium were imported, chiefly by the Portuguese from Goa, the emperor Yung Ching strictly prohibited the sale and smoking of opium. In 1790 the annual report reached 4,000 chests, 16,000 in 1830, more than 25,000 in 1838, and 70,000 in 1858. The consumption of opium rapidly increased to considerable proportions, together with the smuggling of opium, against which new measures were taken in 1820. The last prohibition of the import of opium into China dates from that year. The English, thinking this detrimental to their commerce, the Opium War broke out, beginning by the destruction, on the part of the Chinese, of 20,000 chests of opium, and continuing from 1834 to 1842. The Chinese had finally to purchase peace at the cost of considerable losses in money and territory. Fifteen years later a second war broke out which likewise ended unsuccessfully for China. The Treaty of Tientsin legalized the Chinese opium traffic.[10] In this dire necessity China decided to cultivate the poppy herself. Large tracts of land were devoted to this purpose, at the expense of the cultivation of foodstuffs. In the meantime the passion for opium-smoking had seized on large sections of the population, and was probably augmented by the increased facility for obtaining the drug in the country itself.

A further change took place in 1906. After a century of demoralization through opium, China decided to give up the cultivation of the poppy. According to a convention with England, poppy-growing was to be gradually diminished during a period of ten years, while England was to reduce her opium imports into China at a corresponding rate. The year 1917 marked the end of this agreement, which shows some degree of success. The cultivation of opium ceased in one province after another and the English imports were officially discontinued. But unfortunately, China has no means of controlling the traffic in the foreign concessions, for instance Shanghai, Hong-Kong, and Macao. Here and in other places the Chinese can procure opium and even resell it. Opium for smoking is prepared in Macao. As it is impossible under existing circumstances to introduce it openly into China, it can only be distributed as contraband. Naturally a large quantity is consumed in the town itself in the notorious opium dens where, as I have seen in other places, those possessed with the opium demon lie on the bunks placed one above the other, like the bread-shelves in a bakery, and taste the greatest joy of their earthly lives.

If it is asked what becomes of the large amount of opium produced in British India, for instance in Patna, Malwa, Benares, we may consider it more than probable that it reaches China by indirect routes.

This opium, produced in the United Provinces, is Monopoly-Opium. The whole yield must be delivered to a Government agent at a fixed price. It is then sent to the State factory at Ghazipur to be rendered suitable for the market. Every month auctions of this substance take place at Calcutta. The product obtained in the native states of Rajputana and Central India, which is subject to duty on entering the British area, realizes the same price as English opium.

Recent information[11] shows that during the last few years large amounts of Indian opium of enormous value have been accumulating at the free ports outside the naval customs barrier. In the year 1912 the value of opium deposited at Shanghai alone was estimated at £11,000,000 sterling. According to the agreement it cannot be imported into China until there is proof that opium is being cultivated in China itself. The great efforts which China has made in order to obtain her deliverance from opium have caused millet and cotton to spring up even in the most distant corners of the empire, where formerly stretched many-coloured fields of poppies. This beneficial policy seems now to be meeting with certain obstacles. The savage tribes of Eastern Tibet, although for the greater part independent, are nevertheless included in the Chinese territory according to the terms of the opium convention. In the solitude of isolated and inaccessible mountains far from the world, in places to which Chinese authority and its agents penetrate rarely and with difficulty, these tribes cultivate the poppy and introduce its juice surreptitiously into China. It is remarkable that the Chinese were unable to impart the passion for opium to the aborigines in Central Tibet to any greater extent.

Latterly Japan has been the greatest buyer of opium in Calcutta.[12] The merchandise arrives at Kobe and is thence conveyed to Tsingtao. Very considerable quantities of morphia are said to be manufactured in Japan, which are sold in Manchuria by Japanese merchants bearing Formosa passports. From Tsingtao it is conveyed via the provinces of Shantung, Nganhwei, and Kiangsu; from Formosa, together with opium, to Fokien and Kwang-tung. In this way China is deliberately overrun from this side with these two products. The total quantity is estimated at 20 tons a year. An injection of morphia costs 3 to 4 cents.

The export of morphia to the Far East from England increased up to 1914 (see Table 1).

TABLE 1. EXPORT OF MORPHIA TO THE FAR EAST FROM ENGLAND	
YEAR	AMOUNT OF MORPHIA EXPORTED
1911	5 $\frac{1}{2}$ tons
1912	7 $\frac{1}{2}$ tons
1913	11 $\frac{1}{4}$ tons
1914	14 tons

According to information from Japanese sources the export of morphia from England fell from 600,229 ounces in 1917 to a quarter of this amount in 1918; this is to be explained by the manufacture of this product in Japan itself.

What this new "morphia-phase" in the history of opium means for the population of the Far East, if, as is certain, morphia should continue its triumphant march, can be gathered from our experience of this drug in Europe. It is already reported that there were numerous victims of morphinism in the years 1914 and 1915.

It is related that years ago an old opium smoker earnestly desired to be broken of the unfortunate habit. He offered a large reward for a cure. One of his compatriots, who had learnt the use of morphia from a foreign physician, offered to cure him, and treated him with injections of morphia. The sensations which the opium-smoker experienced were so agreeable that he very soon abandoned his opium-pipe. The quack went to Hong-Kong and proclaimed that he possessed an unfailing remedy for the opium habit. In a short time the number of his clients increased to such an extent that he erected a whole series of institutions for the injection of morphia. At last there were about twenty in existence. Finally the government ordered the closing of these establishments for human destruction and prohibited the supply of morphia without a doctor's prescription. Now this evil continues to develop clandestinely.

Such Indian opium as does not reach China by a direct route seeks for other markets, and reaches Chinese merchants and consumers through indirect channels. Those Chinese territories which are in foreign possession import particularly large quantities of opium. In the foreign quarters of Shanghai the number of opium shops increased

from 131 in 1908 to 663 in 1916. The inhabitants of the Chinese
quarter can obtain any amount from these shops. The situation is the
same in Hong-Kong, Kowloon, and Liangtua.

Next to India, Turkey and Persia are the greatest producers of
opium in the world. A large part of the Persian opium, called in its
pure state Shire-Teriak, but when adulterated for export and consumption Teriak-i-Chume and Teriak-i-Jule, goes to Hong-Kong and
Formosa and from there probably to China also. This is probably the
reason why it is not included in the following table of the countries of
origin of opium. Opium is cultivated through Persia. The best qualities are supplied, among other places, by Isaphan and Shiraz—also
famous on account of its wine—Shiraz, the valley of roses and night-
ingales, which shelters the tombs of the poets Hafiz and Saadi. Isaphan
is the center of the opium trade. So long as forty years ago 2,000 boxes
of opium, representing a value of about £ 150,000, were exported from
Bushire to England.

Large quantities of opium are now produced also in Macedonia,
Bulgaria, and Yugoslavia. The last-named country before the war produced annually an average of about 120,000 kilos. It has lately increased to 150,000 kilos, representing a value of 200 million dinars.

In Egypt the cultivation of opium is prohibited.

Other countries also import considerable quantities, for instance,
Cochin-China, which imported in 1912–13 840 chests of opium each
of 140 pounds, in 1914–15 2,690, and in 1916–17 3,440 chests.

In Saigon crude opium, which is a State monopoly, is refined into
smoking opium, or chandu. Already twenty years ago 67,000 kilos of
crude opium were annually refined to 44,800 kilos of chandu. The
annual consumption of opium, without counting contraband, is estimated at 120,000 kilos. The smokers were mainly the Chinese living
in centers such as Saigon or Cholon. Considerable quantities are delivered to distant parts. The small island of Mauritius, for instance,
imported in 1912–13 only ten chests, but in 1916–17 as many as 120.

Table 2 illustrates Germany's position with regard to opium, and
also shows the countries of origin of the drug.

TABLE 2. IMPORTS OF OPIUM INTO GERMANY								
COUNTRY OF ORIGIN	AMOUNTS IN DOUBLE-CENTNERS (100 KG)							
	1911	1912	1913	1920	1921	1922	1923	1924	1925
Greece	4	14	15	34	225	230	60	45	182.1
Switzerland	—	—	—	78	—	21	12	74	98
Turkey	638	504	754	500	410	1314	1286	599	904
British India	84	19	278	—	14	19	26	77	—
China	103	141	64	8	43	156	18	21	24.84
United States	—	—	—	5	47	118	—	13	—
Yugoslavia	—	—	—	—	—	—	—	—	57
Total	1040	868	1625	787	790	1906	1409	841	1507

The Consumption of Opium and Morphia at the Present Day

An alarming spectacle is presented to the observer who undertakes to describe the extension of the passion for opium and morphia from a scientific point of view. Morphia, a scourge of recent date, has established itself all over the world. It is always ready for use, and can be taken simply and conveniently without any elaborate apparatus: a syringe, a small flask, and a dark corner is all that is needed. The arm or thigh can be pierced with the needle through the clothes; no odour reveals the dope victim, as in the case of opium, no drowsiness to necessitate lying in a horizontal position—the absorption of the morphia solution in the subcutaneous tissues has the power to transform the individual who was tortured by abstinence and unable to work into a hero ready to cope with the exigencies of modern life. The time will come—if no miracle happens—when the more recent drug, morphia, will have at least unthroned if not vanquished its ancient and clumsy rival, opium. Nevertheless, there will always be some who seek a life of dreams and visions, such as the smoking of opium produces, who will prefer the latter drug because its effects are more attractive and alluring than the cold action of morphia. That is why even in our days isolated devotees of opium are to be found all over Europe. It is not long since the discovery that the drug was taken in Paris in certain places by women, even young girls. Just before the war the Chamber of Deputies and French public opinion were stirred by the revelation that in the French navy and particularly in the naval ports in the Mediterranean opium-smoking had developed to a degree dangerous to the whole nation. A part of the opium was said to originate from the State factories in Indo-China; the rest was of European origin.

There are other countries in Europe where decrepit and degenerate habitués of both sexes, men and women of the demi-monde, victims of a violent and blind craving for sensation, are addicted to smoking opium. The farther east we go, the larger the number of opium maniacs. The opium habit obtains in the Balkans and increases as we approach Asia Minor. In some places, for instance in Damascus, it is clandestinely indulged in, but as an acknowledged drug it has permeated all social ranks. Of the three Iranian countries, Baluchistan, Afghanistan, and Persia, the last-named occupies an important rank among opium-consuming lands. In the northern provinces, particularly in Khorasan, both Mohammedans and non-Mohammedans smoke a great deal of opium. Bokhara and Afghanistan consume only a small amount. But many a heavy consignment has doubtless crossed the Hindu-kush and the frozen passes leading to Eastern Turkestan. Here, for instance in Kashgar, men and women avidly smoke opium in publicly recognized opium dens.

Farther south, towards India, the passion for opium increases. In the states of Rajputana the hardiest native races, the Rajputs and Sikhs, smoke opium, and the Hindus also are addicted to this vice. On the coast of Coromandel all social classes make use of the opium pipe, the Hookah. A mixture of opium and rose-leaves is smoked with a little tobacco. There are also opium eaters, for instance in Bengal. Some years ago the number of opium addicts in Hyderabad, out of a population of eleven million, was estimated at over one million, including 12 per cent Mohammedans, 7 per cent Hindus, and 5 per cent Pariahs, people from the towns and the plains as well as from the highlands. Opium-eating is taboo among some religious sects, e.g. the Yeragis in Eastern Bengal. The ratio of men to women among the opium-eaters of India is approximately 73:27. They are for the most part thirty to forty years of age.

In the territories of Rajputana, Central India, and the province of Gujarat during festivals a 5 per cent solution of opium is used, called amalpani or kusamba. The smoking of opium is practiced almost exclusively in the cities. Extracts of opium are used under the names of maddak and chandu, the latter being an extremely concentrated extract which is consumed after a maturation process lasting twelve months under the influence of *aspergillus niger*.

The chain of opium-using countries continues to the south of the Himalayas as far as the territory around the Brahmaputra. In Assam the natives have given themselves up completely to opium. The Kachari are so passionately addicted to it that they demand to be paid in opium instead of money. Both men and women among the Kakhyens, Karens, and Lapais, the inhabitants of the Kasi mountains, smoke opium. They can cultivate only very small quantities on account of the height of the mountains, and they obtain the greater part from China. The savage Turungs and Nagas descend from their hills into the valleys in order to barter ivory, cotton, etc., for rice and opium. The craving for the drug increases eastwards towards the China Sea, and both here and in the Pacific Ocean takes the form of a vital necessity. Certain tribes of Burma, the Pa-yii and the Kachin, smoke opium as their principal occupation. The powerful force of imitation does not spare Siam. In spite of the severest penalties, opium has forced its way via Mekong to Tonkin, Annam, Cambodia, and Cochin-China. The Tonkinese smoke less than the Cochinese, especially the upper classes. Among these, as among the Annamese, who are reputed to be hysterical as a result of opium, a moderate smoker consumes 60 to 80, a heavy smoker up to 150 pipes a day.

An extensive contraband trade in Chinese opium also exists in these parts. It is cheaper than that supplied by the local French agents in Saigon, Hanoi, etc., and unfortunately many Europeans are to be found among the buyers.

The most diverse physical disturbances afflict the opium-smoker; among others, peculiar inflammations of the mouth, stomach disorders and disturbances of the circulatory system, heart diseases, weakness of the limbs resembling paralysis, and occasionally also disturbances of the bladder. With respect to the activity of the brain the same disorders can be observed with which morphinists are afflicted.

We now come to the country where the consumption of opium is greatest—China. This is also the centre from which Chinese emigrants have carried the opium vice with them throughout the world. Far away from their home country the Chinese have transported this habit; along the Manchurian railway, deep in the immense forests, only accessible by narrow paths, small farms for the cultivation of poppies can be found. The opium from these is secretly sold in the towns, particularly in Harbin.

Wherever the opium habitué turns his steps, the drug accompanies him. It follows him into civilization, to America, Canada, Vancouver Island, Alaska, Africa, Australia.

In China itself opium is smoked to an excessive degree. There is hardly a province which is an exception to this rule. In Chinese Turkestan the Shantu are addicted to opium. In Kan-Su, in the southern Kulu-nor country, it has been estimated that 80 per cent of the population of the towns and 30 to 40 per cent in the villages smoke the drug, and that their approximate monthly ration is from 150 to 200 gr. per head. Tafel on his expedition through Tibet encountered hardly anyone who did not smoke opium. Yunnan and Szechwan are the provinces whose population suffers most from this scourge. The missionaries of Kiang-Si complain of the smoking of opium, and especially of the eating of the drug by women, this latter being tantamount to suicide. Throughout the vast territories of the Chinese empire the traveller may witness the disastrous effects which opium has exercised and will continue to exercise on mankind.

The drug has forced its way into Mongolia. Prshevalsky, who explored China with remarkable success fifty years ago and predicted the disastrous effects the opium plague would have for China, found this drug also in Ala-Shan. The passion for its reigns also in Formosa. Even the chewing of betel by the savage Chinwan has been replaced by the opium habit. In Japan, however, the drug seems to have lost its sway.

Seventy thousand Chinese live in the Philippines, the greater part of them opiomaniacs. Many of the natives are addicted to the vice, which the Spaniards attempted to abolish by a State monopoly of opium. America seeks to remedy the evil by severe punishment, treatment centres, and instruction. But she is unable to prevent the consumption in the homeland.

The use of opium forced its way irresistibly into the Dutch Archipelago, to Java and Sumatra, where the natives of Batavia are passionately addicted to the drug and have attacks of delirium if their supply is suddenly stopped. It reached Nias, the islands of the Banda Sea, the eastern Moluccas and Western New Guinea, the Aru and Key Islands, Ceram and Borneo, where it is not only smoked by the savage Dyaks but also by the Chinese. The trade is a monopoly in the islands of Oceania, as it is also in other parts of the world. Agencies for the sale of the drug are established in the smallest village.

The opium vice of the Chinese has found its way even to the fifth continent, Australia, where it was introduced side by side with alcohol. The Chinese, however, did not derive the main profit therefrom, but they left this to the Europeans. Alcoholism, and still more the smoking of opium, which the natives very rapidly copied from the whites and Chinese, has inspired them with a fatal inclination for "dope" and brought about a remarkable reduction in their numbers. In their camps in Queensland and other parts we can observe the decrepitude and the feeble aspect of the Maoris, formerly a very robust race. For the most part imported opium is employed. Attempts at cultivation have revealed a product of a remarkable quality.

The South Sea islands have also fallen under the spell of opium, that triumphant poison. It remains wherever it has sunk its roots. We have information about conditions on certain of these islands, e.g. the Gilbert and Marquesas Islands. The Chinese brought with them the taste for opium which unfortunately supplanted the harmless kava which had until then been in use. The natives of the Marquesas Islands buy the opium from an agent-general of the French State monopoly, who at the end of the last century was only allowed to sell it to the Chinese.

The opium habit has taken root in those parts of Africa in which poppies are cultivated. This is the case in Egypt, for instance, where its degenerating influence on the lower classes was pointed out many years ago. In Tunis and in the towns along the west part of the north coast of Africa opium is only smoked clandestinely and to a very small extent. In the Tripolitan town of Mursuk more users of the drug can be found. In Arabia the smoking of opium has developed hardly at all. In Mecca there is a street named "Kashkarshia,"[13] i.e. street of the opium-sellers.

The customers descend into a kind of empty cellar wherein ledges for sitting are provided along the wall. Men can be found there with a pale and bloodless appearance in spite of their brown skin. Everyone has a small pipe in his hand and inhales the smoke of the glowing opium, which is condensed on the moist mucous membrane of the respiratory passages. All the smokers are silent. From time to time one or another of them ejaculates "O Allah," or "O divine goodness!" In East and Central Africa, for instance near Mazaro on the banks of the Kwakwa in Mozambique, the Hindus from Malwa organized poppy cultivation several years ago. The use of opium, however, in that region is not considerable. Not many Arabs have been brought by the Hindus to the smoking of opium. In other parts, for instance in East Africa, in Uganda, or on the banks of the Congo, only the Chinese workmen smoke.

The extension of the use of opium in the United States of America is of very great interest, especially on account of the war declared by the legislature in that country against alcohol. Reports published over thirty years ago tell of the increase of the use of opium in some districts, for instance Albany. Whereas the population increased by 59 per cent, the consumption of opium increased by 900 per cent, and that of morphia by 1,100 per cent. It was generally alleged that the largest increase took place in the prohibition states. Recent statistics disclose facts which testify only too clearly to the alarming growth of this evil.

According to statements made by the Chief Medical Officer of New York City in 1921, the Americans consume twelve times as much opium as any other people in the world. More than 750,000 pounds are imported annually into the States, that is, 2.5 gr. per head of the population. The amount of opium used for legitimate purposes does not amount to more than 70,000 pounds a year. The report of a physician of the great New York State prison proves the increase of opiomania in the capital. The number of persons convicted of illegal consumption of opium increased by 789 per cent in the years 1918 to 1921. I do not establish any relationship between these figure, which I do not question, and the prohibition of alcohol. There are many opinions on the prohibitionist side which partly dispute the increase in the number of drug-takers, or, if it must be conceded, give other reasons for it.

What I have outlined above proves emphatically that neither the world's broadest oceans not its highest mountains can serve as a defence against opium and morphia, those drugs which enslave the human brain, enervate the mind, and force the body to follow vices which are fatal to its existence.

An attempt to remedy this calamity is almost certainly doomed to failure. Even if the smoking-dens of the Far East were completely abolished, it would not be possible to suppress the vice in the home. And what is more unfortunate, morphia and the morphia syringe will always be employed.

What is taking place in the Far East, where the injection of morphia is replacing the opium pipe, clearly shows that if it was impossible to suppress the old evil it will be all the more impossible to control the new vice which is developing. This is all the more true, perhaps, because the distribution of the drug by traders cannot be effectively checked. In the Spring of this year some merchants were prosecuted in Hamburg for having diverted to China about 50 kilos of morphia after a permit had been issued for their export to Turkey.

There are also many curious means employed in Germany for inducing people to the consumption of opium. In 1918 it was officially stated in Würtemberg that the use of the stalks and capsules of poppies was being openly recommended as a substitute for tobacco, and that these were in consequence purchased for this purpose. The capsules of poppies in a ripe or unripe state contain enough opium to produce the effects of the drug if inhaled as smoke.

Morphinism

Morphia very early commenced its triumphant march in Europe. The span is short that separates its discovery in 1817 from the year 1830, when Balzac, that keen observer of human nature, in his *Comédie du diable* makes the devil enumerate the reasons why he has no time to seek his personal pleasure. What hinders him is the enormous increase in the population of his kingdom, hell, as a result of the discovery of gunpowder, printing, morphia, etc. At that time, indeed, morphia served mainly as a suicidal agent. Very soon, however, morphiomania supervened. It increased mysteriously to an extent which very few foresaw, and the number of its slaves gradually augmented. The great wars of the epoch, the Crimean War and its successors, contributed to its development. Not long after I had reported a case of morphinism in a ward attendant in 1874, the first curative treatment was undertaken. The extension of the evil, which until then had been hidden, became apparent.

The causes of its development were and are those I have already indicated:

(1) The impossibility of breaking away from the morphia habit after it has served as an anodyne and anæsthetic. The sensation of extreme well-being experienced on such an occasion enslaves the person to its further use, although the initial cause has disappeared.

(2) The desire to be freed from a state of depression or mental excitement.

(3) Curiosity and the instinct of imitation, soon leading to the pure and simple desire for a euphoric state which in due time makes the individual a slave to the drug. Among medical men the idea existed for a long time that they could not become addicted to the drug. Experience has proved the contrary. A large number of doctors are morphinists. A statistical table of addicts, including all countries of the world, gave 40.4 per cent doctors, and 10.0 per cent doctors' wives.

In Paris the number of morphinists was estimated at 50,000, that is, one to every forty inhabitants. At the present day this figure is said to have considerably increased. Many years ago I pointed out that if alcohol ruins the hands of the people, morphia ruins their heads. Actually, during the last few decades and especially after the Great War, morphinism has developed in the former direction also. But medical men, professors, pharmacists, writers, artists, lawyers, officers, high officials etc., still predominate among this class of drug-takers.

The demoniac power of morphia can even be established among animals. I administered the drug to pigeons daily at a certain time. The effect of the injections abated within a few hours and the birds remained in their cages in a state of depression; but as soon as I approached with the syringe they came out, flapping their wings.

A cat was injected daily with morphia during a longer period. After some time it was apathetic before the injections. After treatment this state was reversed. After thirty-four days the animal died from emaciation on account of digestive disorders. The avid desire for opium was also established in the case of a monkey. Very far down in the animal kingdom, in rats, etc., and even in bees, the violent craving for opium or poppies has been observed. In the countries where opium is smoked, cats, dogs, and monkeys inhale the smoke which their master expels from his opium-pipe, and it is said that monkeys consume the opium which oozes from the bamboo pipe.

Infants can also be habituated to opium. A child of four months whom the nurse provided with decoctions of opium capsules in increasing quantities for insomnia, was cheerful when waking from sleep and readily took the bottle. It pined away as soon as withdrawal of the drug was attempted, and the application of the beverage had to be prolonged. After a further two-and-a-half months the child died. Its physical and intellectual development had not made the least progress during this lapse of time. Visual and auditory perceptive faculties were hardly observable; the child recognized nobody and had a fixed stare.

The evil practice, to give it no worse name, of doping children with decoctions of opium or tincture of opium in doses which must necessarily be increased in order to soothe them is widespread and has many victims.

The report of the Royal Commission on Opium, published in several volumes in 1896, contains various misconceptions which are liable to create false impressions. It states, e.g., that the moderate habitual use of opium, which in reality amounts to 0.15–0.8–2.5 gr. per day among 5 to 7 per cent of the population of India, is quite harmless to the well-being of and the health of the people, on account of the power of resistance of the Hindu to this toxic agent. The custom of giving opium to children in order to keep them quiet and to enable the mother to carry on her work undisturbed, a custom which obtains in the states of Rajputana and Malwa and in the Bombay presidency, the report likewise regards as inoffensive. In these countries an initial dose of 3–5 milligrammes is administered in the first weeks or months of the young life, and is gradually increased to 15–30 milligrammes, and even to 0.12 gr. once or twice a day. In Bombay "Pills for Children" (Bala-Golis) are sold which contain 0.01–0.02 gr. of opium. After the children have reached the age of two to five years they are weaned from opium. How this is done is not described. Deaths from excessive doses do not occur among Indian children, but "only" sometimes dysentery, whereas European children treated in the same way by their nurses are apt to die. In these reports the facts are correct but the conclusions are wrong.

Morphinistic mothers bear morphinistic children who are restless and excitable, and can only be soothed by opium. Suckling with the milk of a morphinistic mother is liable to produce a drug habit in the child, because the morphia passes into the milk.

Family morphinism is particularly tragic, the wife and even the children being lured to the drug-habit by the father. It is impossible to explain the psychological impulse which leads the original drug victim to commit such an act. If mental disease were not taken into consideration it would constitute a crime according to our moral code. For every morphinist knows or will learn that his passion will compel him to follow a path of misery to the bitter end. If it were not for his intellectual disturbance he would, by offering a chronic poison to others, be knowingly thrusting them into disaster. The fact that this takes place with the victims' consent does not mitigate the offence.

The possibility of keeping up an appearance of normality and of continuing to lead within certain limits an ordinary life, exists, as I have already stated, by the gradual increase of the doses of the drug as demanded by the cells of the individual brain. The daily consumption, which at the beginning was a few centigrams, may increase to 4 to 5 gr. Even in the case of infants it is necessary to augment the initial dose. A child of seven months with hydrocephalus received 0.2 milligramme a day. The dose had to be increased to 0.6 gr., which after eight and a half months occasioned death.

The ever-menacing and perpetually increasing internal lassitude of the brain, incessantly roused by the drug to a certain degree of activity, finally gains the victory. The last very large doses of morphia have toxic effects only, and scarcely permit their normal activity to the brain and the organs under its direction. The extent of time occupied by this process varies with the individual, i.e. according to his internal powers of resistance. Every prognosis may collapse before the varying and incalculable possibilities of the vital activity of an individual life.

We are entirely cut off from all knowledge of the internal process which takes place during the use of morphia. We can only perceive the phenomena. It is in vain that we ask for an explanation. It is a subject on which meditation is fruitless and always ends in an admission of our inability to comprehend it. Psychology has so far avoided investigation in the field of the abnormal mental activity produced by the use of narcotics, except in the case of *anhalonium lewinii*. It is more than doubtful whether the most exhaustive analytical experiments will ever produce positive results. It will, in my opinion, never be ascertained why the brain-cells exhibit such a violent craving for morphia (which in the case of alcohol is less apparent) and why the strongest resolution of the morphinist fades to nothing before the imperative demand of the brain-cells.

The Observable Internal Process in Morphinists and Opiumists

The effects of the prolonged use of morphia unfold themselves in several stages which cannot be accurately separated but have each their particular character. The beginning of the process finds the morphinist in a state of delusion with regard to the value of his faculties, his work, and his agreeable sensations. The ego bases itself on a false valuation with respect to the personality itself and the rest of the world. But whatever be the cause of this psychological change, the individual himself perceives it, work seems to progress more favorably, the small buffets that life dispenses are not felt as such, and this increased vitality lasting six to eight hours is the result of one dose of morphia.

This introductory, seductive stage, which may extend over a period of months, is succeeded on increasing the dose by the more delicious second morphinistic period, filled with a feeling of well-being, absolute contentment, free from desire, undisturbed mental calm.

An opium-eater who arrived at this stage has expressed his sensations in an emphatic style which we must consider as corresponding to his real impressions: "O just, subtle, and all-conquering opium! that, to the hearts of rich and poor alike, for the wounds that will never heal, and for the pangs of grief that 'tempt the spirit to rebel,' bringest an assuaging balm . . . thou buildest upon the bosom of darkness, out of the fantastic imagery of the brain, cities and temples, beyond the art of Phidias and Praxiteles . . . and 'from the anarchy of dreaming sleep' callest into sunny light the faces of long-buried beauties . . . Thou only givest these gifts to man; and thou hast the keys of Paradise."

The flood of the obstacles of life breaks on the morphinized brain without leaving any impression or trace. No disagreeable mental state is felt as a discomfort; care or sorrow hardly touch the soul. Lighter emotion such as worry and indignation evaporate without making any

impression at all. Freed from everything which ties man to earth, free
even from the feeling of possessing a body, the individual lives consciously, with open eyes, a life of dreams. This life, however, is a purely
"ego" life, a life in the present. The thoughts are directed not to the
future but only to the passing day with its morphia. Soon the higher
perceptions become defective. Heart and soul suffer. The limitation
of the world to oneself causes moral deterioration and renders the
individual ruthless even towards wife and children. His care for the
latter, if present at all, is quite secondary to the craving anxiety for
morphia. The poet's words[14] are in a figurative sense true:

> Zur Warnung hört' ich sagen,
> Dass, der im Mohne schlief,
> Hinunter ward getragen
> In Träume schwer und tief;
> Dem Wachen selbst geblieben
> Sei irren, Wahnes Spur,
> Die Nahen und die Lieben
> Hält er für Schemem nur.

The duration of action of a single dose, which now amounts to
0.2–0.5 gr., rapidly diminishes. The drug must be inject more frequently
and in larger quantities, the chain of slavery becomes shorter and tugs
at the morphinist. His creditors, the brain cells, grow restive, demand
satisfaction, shriek, and revenge themselves by producing pain if they
are not satisfied quickly enough. If money to buy the drug is lacking,
he steals or embezzles. Respectable women are said to become prostitutes in order to be able to buy morphia. At the beginning of the
passion for morphia one pleasure is replaced by another still more
delightful, but now a state supervenes wherein the brain after an injection reacts as before, but between two doses, if it is not immediately satisfied, makes its presence very disagreeably felt as soon as the
effect of the last dose begins to pass away.

The passage of time gives birth amid excruciating pains to the last
stage; the awakening to consciousness of the fact that the morphinist
is given over body and soul to the drug, that he has unconditionally
surrendered. Will-power is completely paralysed. Even the effort of
will needed to carry out the simplest act is now lacking. The perpetual
fight between the necessity for decision and the incapacity for it, as

well as the consciousness of inferiority and misery with which the victim is obsessed, cause terrible suffering. Even in his dreams this mental torture is continued, for the happy, delightful past is brought into tormenting comparison with the despair of the present. It is not possible to face each day's work without exaggerated doses of the drug. Its aid enables the morphinistic surgeon to strengthen his trembling hand, to clear his dim eye and his obscured judgment—I have seen this terrible condition in one of the most capable surgeons of the day who had done the work of a genius in his time. The rider can win the race, the judge can pronounce a just judgment, but the will-power, scourged into activity, soon fades away. If the brain is not completely sodden with the drug, compulsory abstinence brings about mental and physical restlessness, inconsiderateness towards others, especially dependents. Many pages might be filled with the description of these symptoms. We could tell of morphinistic judges who in this state deal unjustly with the accused, of high officials who vent the nervous troubles caused by abstinence on their subordinates; even of a professor, long since dead, who could not treat humanely the student he was examining unless his attendant, who was bribed by the students, had some morphia syringes in readiness for him.

In the case of such persons every contact with the higher sentiments, love of the family, good humor, faith, reverence, the beauty of nature and the activities of human life is lost, and that forever. The sunny side of existence, which even in the case of the most poor and desolate being possessed of a clear brain brings some moments of subjective satisfaction and happiness, never lightens the darkness surrounding the morphinist at this stage. Only the picture of long-lost hours of ecstasy remains framed by repentance in his memory. The regret for the life which has been lost is the *Miserere* of annihilation.

As a consequence of the disorder of the brain-functions organic troubles gradually appear. The brain, the regulating center of so many diverse organs, is slowly but surely paralyzed. Nutrition suffers, the general appearance is bad, emaciation sets in and the capacity for work is greatly reduced. Morphia is able to enforce physical labor only in toxic doses.

During this period the morphinist generally consists of little more than skin, bone, and palpitating nerves. Sticky sweat is excreted, especially at night, from the whole body or from the head alone; the

appearance and personal hygiene are neglected. Frequently attacks of
fever with ague, headache, and oppression occur. There is a tormenting itching of the skin. Gastric pains, colic, diarrhœa with the sore-
ness of the anus, probably occasioned by an unknown decomposition
product of morphia; sometimes disturbances of the urinary excretions,
conjunctivitis, lacrymation, disturbances of accommodation and dullness of vision set in.

Sexual life suffers. At the beginning of morphinism the excitability of the sexual functions increased, but now it diminishes to impo-
tence: *Infringit stimulos veneris opium.* The examination of the semen
of a morphinist who had injected 0.3–0.5 gr. of morphia daily for several months, disclosed quite immobile thin spermatozoa which could
not be rendered mobile even by chemical agency. In morphinistic
women disturbances of menstruation amounting to amenorrhœa set
in. If conception takes place the fetus may be born normally or abor-
tion induced. But even in the former case there is a possibility of its
early death by reason of its feeble vitality. The semen or the ovum of
the mother may be morphinized to such an extent that its normal
functioning is injured, as occurs in cases of poisoning by other substances such as lead-poisoning in the case of lead workers, or mercury
and carbon bisulphide poisoning in industry. After birth the child of a
morphinistic mother may exhibit symptoms of the withdrawal of the
drug.

Reduced to this state, the morphinist seeks help. He wishes to be
liberated from the morphia that is killing him. It cannot be predicted
even approximately when this moment will arrive, nor how long the
individual is capable of working, thinking, and living under the toxic
influence, before he forces himself through the gates of a sanatorium.
His miserable existence may last for a long time before he comes to
this decision. The feeling of inability to carry on may appear after
three or six years, or even much later. The morphinist exhausted by
the burden of the drug is nothing more than a ruin, whose crumbling
into a mass of debris can seldom be avoided. It is of no consequence to
the final result whether withdrawal is attempted suddenly or in stages.
In the former case the suffering produced is serious: and excitement of
the hitherto impotent sexual sphere, restlessness, morbid craving for
morphia, violent crises of fury and destructive mania occur, leading
often to delirium and attempted suicide. Besides these symptoms ex-

cruciating pains are felt in various nervous centres; vomiting, diarrhœa, angina pectoris succeeded by cardiac collapse set in for some days. The gradual deprivation of the drug involves after every diminution of the dose a renewed cry on the part of the cerebral cells for the full amount to which they were adapted. In both cases the morphinist may be delivered from immediate desire for the drug, but that is all. About 80 to 90 per cent of these wretched beings, perhaps even more, have relapses. In this figure are also included those who without being treated in a sanatorium have been temporarily freed from their vice by imprisonment.

The use of other narcotic or stimulating drugs as substitutes for morphia merely augments the evil, since both, the old and the new, are then employed at once. A state then appears which I have named "twofold craving." Forty years ago I drew attention to the combined use of several narcotics, for instance that of morphia with chloroform, ether, or cocaine.[15]

General Questions Connected with Morphinism

Morphinism as a state of intellectual constrain is more dangerous than alcoholism. The recognized and approved rules with respect to alcoholism concerning exclusion from or access to situations of responsibility are valid to a far greater extent with respect to morphinism. Both I myself and others after me have insisted on this.

The morphinist is mentally affected to a greater degree than the drunkard. Such a person cannot be left in positions such as those of examiner, judge, public official, etc., where he may exercise an influence over the welfare of his fellow-creatures. Not only their mental aberrations but even their physical inferiority should prohibit morphinistic workers from holding or continuing to hold responsible positions as engine-driver, pointsmen, permanent-way men, etc.

In the advanced stage of morphinism even the capacity for correct judgment is lost. The poison brings about profound changes in the personality. These manifest themselves in permanent disturbances of will-power and activity which are not only opposed to ethical and moral principles but must also be regarded as illegal if the same laws are applied to morphinism as to alcoholism. It was an error of judgment caused by lack of experience of the ways of the world, which led

a French court to declare valid the will of a morphinist who had committed suicide after leaving his fortune to his mistress. The court was
moved to this verdict by the very frequent but foolish argument that
if responsibility is recognized in criminal law this should likewise be
done in civil law. The law, which protects humanity against the drunkard by all kinds of safeguards and punishments, has hitherto ignored
morphinists, cocainists, and other narcomaniacs, because jurists are
not disposed to leave to the medical profession the statement, substantial proof, and solution of medical problems which involve the
relationship between the individual and public order.[16]

The Committee of the League of Nations which deals with the world-
problem of narcomania apparently makes the same mistake, for it has not
to my knowledge secured the aid of a competent medical expert in relation to these matters. Medical men throughout the world should protest
unanimously against decisions in this matter being left to laymen.

In 1925 the draft of the German General Penal code contained a
paragraph entitled "Abuse of Toxic and Inebriant Poisons", and paragraph 341 deals with the "Supply of Inebriant Poisons" as follows:

"Whosoever without permission supplies any person with opium,
morphia, cocaine, or other narcotic inebriant poisons shall be liable
to a term of imprisonment not exceeding two years or to a fine."

This paragraph, which probably was not edited by a medical man,
is in this form an absurdity. According to the text the force of the law
could be directed, for instance, against a person who supplied another
with alcohol, spirit of ether, ether, benzine, ligroine, etc. The sale of
the substances mentioned above is unrestricted, and the person de-
manding them can apply them according to his own free will as "toxic
and inebriant poisons."

The morphinist should not only not be allowed to transact his
own affairs but should also be compulsorily interned in a sanatorium.
Justification for placing him under tutelage[17] can be found in the fact
that he is unable to manage his affairs on account of the state of his
brain and because in many cases he exposes his family to poverty in
order to procure the drug. He should be placed on the same level as
the inveterate drunkard.[18] Morphinism should also be a ground for
divorce. In an advanced stage of intoxication the morphinist becomes
impotent, and this renders him unfit for the responsibilities of marriage. A married morphinist cheats his wife of the happiness of life in

every way. She also has the right to fulfill her physiological destiny. In such unions the husband often, in his consciousness of guilt, tempts his wife to morphinism.

The German courts have come to different decisions as to the irresponsibility of morphinists, cocainists, etc. They have, for example, punished a morphinist who had falsified prescriptions in order to obtain the drug, while acquitting a morphinistic lawyer who embezzled. A man who after being severely wounded in the war had become a morphinist and constantly committed small thefts and frauds in order to procure the drug was also acquitted. Irresponsibility must be admitted in respect of the greater number of offences committed by drug victims. From a toxicological point of view no difference can be established among morally defective but "intellectually intact" morphinists. The one involves the other, even though laymen consider the intelligence of these drug victims quite undisturbed. If life is subjected to the constraint of a morbid passion, a morbid modification of the personality results, to which in many cases paragraph 52 of the existing penal code must be applied.

The most diverse infringements of the law have been alleged to be the result of morphinism. Recently a thief demanded acquittal because he was under the influence of morphia and not fully conscious when committing his crime. A chemist who had escaped from a sanatorium where he had been interned for demorphinization made use of his liberty to commit a sexual murder. He confessed, but stated that he was intoxicated with morphia. The annals of jurisprudence furnish very many instances of illegal acts committed by morphinists. In order to escape from the suffering of the morphia-inflamed ganglia of the brain with which they are afflicted, they break into pharmacies, drug stores, and hospitals, defraud, embezzle, counterfeit prescriptions (this last was once—mildly—punished); or even when supplied with morphia, they may commit crimes against humanity so that the judge has to decide as to their responsibility.

In the series of cerebral disorders which I have described above (which may explain certain abnormal actions) there occur certain states of abnormal mentality which are rare during the normal course of morphinism but frequent as a result of sudden enforced abstinence. Those patients who have lost the ability to differentiate between right and wrong, true and false, may, if they are predisposed, exhibit psychoses which in their symptoms and course bear the character of an acute mania and cannot be distinguished from confusional insanity. In other case the malady is similar in character to paranoia. The variety of the forms of mental disease which may afflict the morphinist, and which have hitherto not been anatomically explained, peremptorily demands such an attitude on the part of the law as I have indicated above.

Paragraph 17 of the new German penal code in preparation—corresponding to paragraph 52 of the old code—provides for an alleviation of the penalty in case of diminished responsibility resulting from morbid disorders of the mental faculties or mental weakness, but makes an exception of persons who voluntarily lose conscious control of their acts by inebriety. Substances causing cerebral disorders other than alcohol are not mentioned. Whether the law will make an exception of voluntary morphinism is questionable.

Measures against the Extension of Morphinism

The ruling classes in all civilized countries are aware of the increasing danger of the abuse of morphia, cocaine, and other narcotics. A deluge of rules and laws has been the result. Nearly all of these are regulations framed round a green table by officials of ministries of health who have no experience whatsoever of this matter. Many of these enactments years ago proved their ineffectiveness and have been discarded. They all aim at restricting the supply of the drugs to purely medicinal uses, at the centralization of the wholesale supply and the strict supervision of pharmacists. According to the German "Opium Law" all medical prescriptions containing opium, morphia, cocaine, or heroin must be preserved by the pharmacist even when the medicine prescribed is not to be repeated. The prescriptions of copies of them have to be preserved and accessible for at least three years. In Prussia a regulation exists penalizing doctors who do not take due care in supervision of nurses and attendants when supplying narcotic remedies. During the Höfle trial I explained how easily morphinists may be created by lack of supervision in these cases. It was disclosed that at that time the strongest narcotics might easily be procured from subordinates in the prison-hospital without any control. I could not but characterize this as the application of the canteen system to these most dangerous drugs. The consequences were inevitable.

In other countries, for instance in England, the pharmacies are subjected to very strict control. Among other things the prescriptions, which must be preserved and copied into a register, are in principle only allowed to be made up once, or, if specified by the physician, up to a maximum of three times. The possession and the illegal use of morphia and cocaine not prescribed by a doctor is punished with imprisonment. In the British Malay States the "Deleterious Drugs Enactment" of September, 1925, exclusively reserves the import and export of the drugs specified in the law to the superior officer of the health department. Physicians and pharmacists can only obtain supplies and procure these drugs through the medium of the medical officers. The law prohibits the manufacture of morphia and cocaine and their salts and the possession of more than twelve legal doses of any narcotic or of preparations thereof, whether for internal or injecting purposes, without permission.

All legislative safeguards may be and are eluded. They are necessary, but we cannot depend upon their strict observance. The passion of the morphinist and the avarice of the dealer, even when the latter is the State itself, break down all barriers. At this final conclusion all those who are acquainted with the facts arrive. With extraordinary effrontery certain proprietary articles are sold (for instance Trivalin) which contain not only morphia but also cocaine. For every thousandth of a gramme of the latter there is a disproportionate increase in the danger of the mixture. Unconscious of the far-reaching consequences of their prescriptions, medical men become accomplices in such mercenary businesses. Other dealers sell morphia wholesale to those who will pay their price. The circumstances guarantee discretion on both sides. Many other proofs could be cited of the difficulties, not to say impossibilities, encountered in the attempt to remedy this evil.

It is difficult to say whether some kind of international State monopoly of these substances, such as has been suggested, would be able to combat this growing menace to mankind and the vile traffic to which it gives rise.

The League of Nations in Geneva may be of help. The discussions of the Opium Conference have up to the present (1925) jeopardized the hopes that were based on the international regulation of the production of and traffic in opium. America, which considers herself commercially disinterested in the subject, proposed a limitation of the production of raw opium and coca leaves in the countries of origin to the quantities necessary for medical and scientific requirements. The aim in view was "to offer a gleam of hope to millions of families who suffer from the consequences of the abuse of opium and other narcotics." India did not agree to such a limitation, and earned the reproach of being influenced in opium politics by financial and commercial considerations. Japan also formulated demands in respect of opium to which India refused to agree. A gradual reduction of the traffic in opium and a simultaneous decrease of the evil for fifteen years were taken into consideration. But this proposal of compromise was also rejected. The Opium Conference has practically broken down. Napoleon once said in the Council of State: "Le commerce n'a pas de patrie." If the activity of commerce in the field of narcotics were characterized properly and plainly, the reproach levelled at it would be a much more serious one.

Finally, I am absolutely certain that no substitute exists which, without containing opium or any of its derivatives, can cure the morphinist of his passion or even alleviate it. All the specifics that have been advertised and sold at high prices with this end in view are based on error or fraud. Years ago a remedy of this kind, of America origin, which was said to contain *piscidia erythrina*, was widely sold under a false name. It contained morphia, and after I had disclosed the fraud, disappeared.

Neither *combretum sundaicum*, nor *mitragyna speciosa* and *mitragyna parvifolia*, the leaves of which are smoked in Perak as "anti-opium," nor *blumea laciniata* can secure a mental calm in the least resembling that obtained from morphia-containing substances, nor maintain a natural combat against the existence of the craving.

In morphia are combined a blessing and a curse. If it is dispensed by the hand of the physician its power is divine. There are human beings who spend sleepless nights in excruciating pain, who because of some disease racking body and soul foresee a morrow and a future covered with a mantle of darkness and night, who curse their life because death will not come, who lead a wretched existence as a result of the destructive powers at work within them, and with certain death in view; to all such the physician should bring the beneficent morphia to alleviate their suffering, to reconcile them to their fate, and to sweeten death. But not to hasten death! He is not authorized to do this, although in morphinism life and death often meet. He should only use the drug in those diseases compared with which morphinism can be regarded as trivial. He should take care not to dispense it injudiciously as an anæsthetic. To do so is to create morphinists who acquire a moral blemish if over and above the anesthetic application they find pleasure in its use, or continue to employ it solely for the purpose of obtaining delightful sensations. Such can expect no mercy, though it must be admitted that they are subject to the constraint of the morphia-craving cerebral cells, which can break down a weakly resistant will-power. Those others alone deserve pity whose life has become a martyrdom into which morphia brings soothing balm. The words of the German physician-poet, inspired by the Muse with deep human sympathy, are true indeed:

Pflücket den Veilchenstrauss, die ihr den Mai ersehnt,
Die ihr geliebt euch wisst, schmückt euch mit Rosenpracht.
Aber des Unglücks Sohn, der nichts sich wünscht als Vergessen,
Wähle den Mohn sich zum Labsal!

Wenn ihn die lange Nacht quälet mit bitterem Schmerz,
Wenn er sich schlaflos wälzt, stöhnend im Folterbett,
Da lang alles entschlief und der Zeiger der pickenden Wanduhr
Stocket im schläfrigen Kreislauf.

O, wie segnet er dich, der Gequälten Trost,
Den heilkundig ein Freund in des Vergessens Trank
Darreicht, wenn ihm das Leid an dem brennenden Auge sich schliesset,
Und die beglückende Gottheit.

Naht auf dem Wagenthron, den ein Eulenpaar
Ohne Geräusch bewegt! Träufle, o träufle, o träufle ihm
Huldvoll perlenden Tau, dass die schmachtende Seele sich labe.
Herrlicher König der Traumwelt!

Zaubre die Jugend vor seinen entzückten Geist,
Lass ihn noch einmal schaun glücklicher Tage glanz,
Maiduft hauch' ihm gelind in die schmerzverdunkelt Seele,
Hoffnung der besseren Zukunft![19]

CODEINE AND ITS DERIVATIVES: DIONINE, HEROIN, EUCODAL, CHLORODYNE

All those substances derived from opium or morphia and containing the morphia nucleus, with names such as Pantopon, Holopon, Glycopon, Laudopan, Nealpon, Eumecon, Trivalin, have in common the property of evoking an ardent desire for their prolonged use. This effect may have less serious consequences than those caused by the original substances; the craving may be less violent, but its action on the individual and the distressing results of compulsory deprivation of the drugs are the same.

Codeine

The widely-used drug codeine is a morphia alkaloid, contained in opium, and is chemically mono-methyl-morphia. To believe that in users of the drug the organism acquires greater ability to destroy it is an error. In dogs 80 per cent of the codeine is excreted with the urine. The conclusion has quite erroneously been drawn from this fact that the drug cannot give rise to a habit because the amount of its destruction in the body, even on prolonged use, is very inconsiderable. It has been said that instead of an habituation to the drug an increased sensibility towards it is manifest. This is an example of the precautions which must be taken in applying to man the results of experiments on animals.

Codeinists have the same abnormal desires, sensations, and sufferings as morphinists. Their number is small in comparison with the latter, but nevertheless considerable. One such, an extremely neuropathic young man, on account of his mental erethism, was prescribed codeine pills, 1 of 0.03 gr. to be taken three times a day. He experienced one day a euphoric state after taking a large number of them at once. He continued to augment the dose, increasing it to 50 pills or nearly 2 gr. of codeine per day. Without these pills life seemed impossible to him. The attempt to escape from this necessity produced depression, restlessness, and weariness of life. After a year 5 pills every hour or two did not suffice him. His restlessness increased. On leaving his bed he travelled purposelessly in street cars and by rail. At last he was consuming 100 pills or nearly 3 gr. of codeine daily. He then procured opium pills, and took that expensive fraudulent preparation

"Anti-morphine," which contains morphia as well as other narcotics. He lost weight considerably, became extremely pale, and talked slowly and hesitatingly. Withdrawal treatment produced, besides the craving for codeine, restlessness, irritability, depression, life-weariness, and physical disturbances. The wretched man sacrificed his fortune of 10,000 marks to this expensive passion.

It is clear that other combinations of codeine may give rise to the effects of addiction in fixed proportion to the amount of codeine they contain. This can be asserted of paracodine, which is said to produce a greater sensation of pleasure than codeine, of eucodine, of codeine-methyl bromide, codeonal, and other substances.

Dionine

Dionine, or ethyl-morphine, acts similarly to codeine and does not lack the property of producing a euphoric state. From it dioninism may result.

Heroin

Uninformed persons have often disputed the possibility of addiction to this drug with evil consequences similar to those of the morphia habit. Such a possibility in fact exists; the substance is exported on a large scale to foreign countries purely for euphoric purposes, and the deprivative cure is accompanied in physically enfeebled heroinomaniacs by grave symptoms. It has even been necessary to permit the further use of the drug to patients who, after consuming only 3 to 5 milligrammes a day for several months, complained during the curative treatment of severe dyspnœa, general fatigue, and violent excitability. Such excitation is one of the two results of the action of this drug and of others of the same series, and to which apparently—in contrast to the narcotic action of the others—no habituation takes place.

Habituation to the narcotic action certainly exists. It is established more slowly than in the case of morphia. It can be explained in my view, which has been universally accepted, by a dulling of the functions of the cells. The euphoric state produced by heroin continues present for a longer time than that of morphia, especially if it is to be injected under the skin. Cases have been reported where the daily dose amounted to 0.6 and even 2.8 gr. The results were mental weakness, general nervous debility, digestive disturbances, pungent odour of the breath, dilation of the pupils, loss of sleep, and above all cardiac weakness. The duration of heroinism until decrepitude supervenes is from six to seven years if the doses administered are large.

The symptoms of withdrawal treatment are more serious than with morphia because the cardiac disorders endanger life. Only morphia and not heroin overcomes this. Heroinists may become morphinists in addition if respiratory disturbances, insomnia, etc., jeopardize the cure.

Eucodal

Eucodal is a chemical derivative of the opium-alkaloid papaverin. It is a narcotic, like morphia and codeine, but is said to be superior in its rapidity of action. Its recommendation as a soporific and substitute for morphia in the treatment of addicts of the latter drug have promoted its use. It exhibits no difference from morphia in its habitual use and the consequences thereof. A doctor who employed it against the cardiac troubles from which he suffered continued its application for over a year, and finally took 0.3 gr. daily and became a slave of the drug. Deprivation was accompanied by weakness of the heart, hysterical crying, extreme irritability, suicidal intentions, excessive craving for eucodal, diarrhœa, loss of appetite, sneezing, ague, etc. After complete withdrawal had been accomplished physical recuperation set in. Nevertheless a strange disposition to egocentricity remained. After only four weeks he had a relapse[20] in spite of all his promises.

The wife of this physician also used eucodal for nervous disorders and strong emotions during a period of ten months. The final doses amounted to 0.15 to 0.2 gr. injected subcutaneously. A cure was accomplished in a week, accompanied by pains in the whole body, diarrhœa, and insomnia, but she soon resumed the habit.

I am sure that if one day the synthesis of opium alkaloids is accomplished, the same characteristics with respect to the addiction and the craving for their use will be ascertained as in the case of morphia.

Chlorodyne

It has frequently been stated that chlorodyne, a patent medicine very much in vogue in England, containing chloroform, ether, morphia, and Indian hemp, gives rise to the phenomenon of habituation with all its consequences. Men and even to a greater extent women have been found to make use of it. Its active substance, even from a moral point of view, is the morphia. The quantities which after gradual progress are finally consumed are considerable. Thirty to 60 gr. a day are not unusual doses, and even 150 gr. may be taken daily. Those who fall victims to this evil behave like morphinists, women sell their husbands' property and steal in order to obtain the drug, and spend large sums on their morbid craving.

COCAINISM

History of Coca and Cocaine

Towards the middle of the sixteenth century the second Council of Lima attempted to restrict the use of coca-leaves by the Peruvians, Chilians, and Bolivians. In canon 120 the drug is described as "a useless object liable to promote the practices and superstitions of the Indians." Political, economic, social, and religious reasons gave rise to this decision. It was arrived at when the use of this substance was extensive and its cultivation was at its height, and partly because coca had contributed, among other causes such as drudgery and malnutrition, to a deterioration of the hygienic condition of the Peruvians. The conquistadors co-operated with the proprietors of mines and plantations; they forced the natives to labor and paid them with coca-leaves. In the years 1560–9 the Government prohibited compulsory labor and the administration of coca because "the plant is only idolatry and the work of the devil, and appears to give strength only by a deception of the Evil One; it possesses no virtue, but shortens the life of many Indians who at most escape from the forests with ruined health. They should therefore not be compelled to labor and their health and lives should be preserved." All these restrictions proved of no avail, and coca became a State monopoly, to pass at the end of the eighteenth century into the hands of private enterprise.

All this relates to that wonderful plant, *erythroxylon coca*, which Francesco Pizarro in the year 1533 found in general use as a euphoric when, setting out from San Miguel's Bay, he penetrated with his troops into the interior of Peru. According to an Indian legend narrated by Garcilaso de la Vega the children of the sun had presented man with the coca leaf after the formation of the empire of the Incas, to "satisfy the hungry, provide the weary and fainting with new vigor, and cause the unhappy to forget their miseries." It is probable, however, that the Indians already cultivated the plant before they formed a federation, and the Incas invented the story of its divine origin in order to reserve it to themselves. They made of it a royal emblem; the queen called herself Mama Cuca, and the priests assisted in upholding the divine honors of the plant by using it in various religious ceremonies. The idols of the time as a sign of divinity were represented with one cheek stuffed with coca leaves. Its use gradually extended to the people, and it was not only applied for supernatural purposes, but for the very worldly object of allowing the plant to act on the organism. Time has changed nothing in this state of affairs, except that the desire for pleasurable sensations now forms the principal motive for the use of the leaves in South America and of cocaine, their derivative, in the rest of the world.

The leaf is chewed mixed with lime or vegetable ashes. The latter, called "lluta" in Aimarà, "llipta" in Keshua, and elsewhere "tonra," are kept in bottle-shaped gourds and extracted with the aid of a needle, the point of which is moistened in the mouth. I possess some preparations which show that these ashes are also found in the form of a circular bluish-gray paste, 4 cm. in diameter, small pieces of which are added to the leaf. Coca is mainly cultivated in Peru in the Montaña in the departments of Cuzco, Huanuco, Ayacucho, and Puno. In all the deep and hot valleys small plantations can be found. The Keshua and aymara tribes in Cundinamarca, etc., are consumers of it. In Bolivia, especially in the departments of Cochabamba, Larecaja, and Yungus, in Colombia up to the Gulf of Maracaibo—the Goajiros are addicts—and to a less extent in Ecuador, but only in some valleys of the east slopes of the Cordilleras of Quito, the habit is in vogue. Its use diminishes as we go farther east from the Andes. It has, however, penetrated slightly along the course of the Marañon. The half-castes and the Indian women of the upper reaches of the Amazon all eat ypadú, as coca is called in those parts. The women plant the shrub, which reaches a height of $1/2$ to $1\,1/2$ metres, in a remote spot of the forest. The Marauá Indians on the banks of the Yutahí, and sometimes the Tecunas, Iuri, Passos, and Yauaretés also partake of the drug. The habit, as Koch-Grünberg observed, seems to have spread from the Rio Tiquié over the Papury. In North-Western Brazil the Indians consume coca in incredible quantities. All day long the calabash passes from hand to hand. Such coca eaters can be seen with lumps in their mouths so that their cheeks protrude like knobs. From Bolivia coca has conquered the Argentine. Peru supplies approximately 15 million, Bolivia 8 million kilos of the leaves which when dry furnish up to 1 per cent cocaine, which is prepared in a raw state in the places of production. In the richest mining district of Peru, in Cerro de Pasco alone, 1,500 kilos of dry coca leaves are consumed monthly. Coca is also cultivated in Java for the manufacture of cocaine. There the tropical sun develops up to 1.2 to 1.6 per cent cocaine in the leaves. In India in the district of the Nilgiris the plant also thrives.

In this case, too, consumption regulates production. The enormous development in the use of the drug explains the increase of the annual export shown in Table 3.

TABLE 3. COCA LEAVES	
PERU	**JAVA**
1877 — 8,000 Kg.	1904 — 26,000 Kg.
1906 — 2,800,000 Kg.	1911 — 740,000 Kg.
1920 — 453,000 Kg.	1912 — 800,000 Kg.
	1920 — 1,700,000 Kg.

The export of raw cocaine increased to the same extent, and for its preparation—according to my personal knowledge—Americans have built large factories in South America.

The cocaine imported into Germany, according to information supplied by the official Bureau of Statistics amounted to 662 kg in 1924 and 1003 kg in 1925.

Effects of the Habitual Use of Coca and Cocaine

The disorders which arise from the habitual use of the coca leaves, which are chewed, and that of cocaine are not the same. The differences are similar to those between opium and morphia. The composition of the two, in fact, is different; in fresh coca leaves there is a fragrant resin and other alkaloids, for instance dextro-cocaine. Experiments which I carried out many years ago with the latter proved that quantities of 0.02 to 0.04 gr. sufficed to produce in rabbits curious mobile excitation; they continuously ran about in circles and were affected by convulsions and respiratory disturbances.

Nevertheless the use of the leaves and that of cocaine produce very similar results as regards the actual symptoms and final form of the cocaine evil.

Coca is for the coca-eater the source of his greatest delight. Under its influence the troubles of life are forgotten and he experiences in imagination many of the substantial pleasures which reality refuses to give. After breakfast and before going to work he takes some coca from his leather bag and some lime or ashes from his gourd and moulds a fragment, and sometimes lays up a stock of these small lumps. Between 25 and 50 gr. is a moderate daily consumption. While chewing he strives to remain idle. An apathetic feeling of internal peace, from which he cannot be awakened, overcomes him for about an hour. Then he is again capable of work.

The cocada, i.e. the duration of the effects of the coca fragment, is his measure of time and distance. It amounts to approximately 40 minutes, during which time about 3 kilometres can be walked or climbed on the plains and 2 kilometres in hilly districts. Alexander von Humboldt, who explored the Andes in 1802, spoke highly of the degree of endurance which his native guides derived from coca. In recent times European explorers have ascertained by experiment on themselves that the ascent to altitudes of 5,000 to 6,000 metres is considerably facilitated by coca, and that thanks to the drug the impression of hunger is not felt for a long time by the ill-conditioned body suffering from malnutrition. Experiments carried out years ago in Europe proved that the drinking of an infusion of 12 gr. of the leaves occasioned, besides a greater frequency of the pulse, palpitation of the heart, faintness, seeing of sparks and *tinnitus aurium*, a feeling of augmented power, and a greater desire for activity. An infusion of 16 gr. of the leaves produced first a strange feeling of isolation from the exterior world and an irresistible urge to use one's strength; then in full consciousness appeared a kind of rigidity with a feeling of the most intense well-being, accompanied by the desire not to make the least movement for the whole day. Finally sleep supervened.

Such was our knowledge of the effects of coca when, in 1885, its active element, cocaine, was introduced into medical science. At that time a morphinistic physician put forward the unfortunate theory that morphinism could be cured by cocaine. I at once objected, predicting that the only result would be the simultaneous use of both drugs, which I called "twofold craving."[21] This, and even worse, is what in fact happened. Cocaine was soon used by itself as a pleasure-producing agent. At first the doses were small, but they increased up to 1 and 4 gr. and it is said that they even reached the enormous dose of 8 gr. a day. To believe that this is due to the war is an error; it has only added to the number of addicts whose social position had hitherto kept them isolated from its influence. Already in 1901 there were many cocainistic men and women in England, doctors, politicians, and writers. At present the situation is evidently much worse, although morphinism has not been dethroned. In Germany, mainly in the large towns, there are many cocainists in every profession, down to prostitutes and their protectors. In certain bars and restaurants, in the street, etc., cocaine is clandestinely sold; very frequently it is stolen or adulterated merchandise for which huge prices up to 30 marks are asked and paid. In Berlin there are cocaine dens, both disreputable and dirty and also fashionable and up-to-date establishments. One of these was raided by the police at the beginning of the present year. About one hundred habitués, men and women, from all classes of society, even university and literary men, had gathered there, to lead for a few hours an existence of somnolence and unreality. They spent whole days without taking food, for cocaine anæsthetizes the nerves of the stomach, thus preventing the appearance of any feeling of hunger. They give all that they possess, even indispensable articles of clothing, in order to indulge their mad craving. The most fantastic descriptions of the night side of human life, the sketch of Hogarth representing a party of punch drinkers, and like works which show the vileness of the human individual at a level below that of the beasts, cannot equal in horror the picture of degradation by such an assembly in the throes of cocaine.

Cocainomania and its Forms

The possibility of the formation of a habit, even to the extent of very large doses of the plant or the alkaloid if they are progressively increased, the obligation of continuing their use, the agreeable sensations which they produce, and finally the physical and moral misery which results from them; such are the evils which are united in cocainomania, as in morphinism and opium-eating. It is remarkable that as opposed to morphia animals cannot become accustomed to cocaine; they even exhibit an increasing sensibility to the drug. The case is, however, on record, of a monkey which became a cocaine-eater through imitation. Perhaps this can be explained by the anthropoid nucleus. The animal searched the pockets and the cupboards of its mistress for cocaine, which it voraciously consumed. The consequences were the same as in man. Leaving this case out of consideration the tolerance of animals towards cocaine shows that this substance has a quite different character from morphia. Its effects on man confirm this opinion from every point of view. Its action on the brain is very much more violent. A single injection into the gums or under the skin may cause serious troubles of the functions of the brain, for instance mental disorders, illusions and melancholia, which appear after one day and frequently last for weeks or months. The prolonged toxicomaniac abuse brings about by gradual development graver symptoms, the manifestations whereof are apparent among those eager coca-eaters of South America, the Coqueros. Physically and morally they behave like opium-smokers. A cachectic state appears with extreme emaciation accompanied by a gradual change of demeanour. They are old men before they are adult. They are apathetic, useless for all the more serious purposes of life, subject to hallucinations, and solely governed by the one passionate desire for the drug, besides which everything else in life is of inferior value.

The use of cocaine has consequences which are much more marked and typical, although they present the same character. The method of its introduction into the body is of no importance. There is no other substance which has so many different modes of application. It may be injected subcutaneously, drunk as a beverage in the form of coca wine, cocaine wine or champagne, smoked in cigarettes, thrust into the nose with a brush or employed as snuff, rubbed into the gums or the anus. Every method has its followers. It seems that the greatest number prefer the nasal cavity as the place of application.[22] Out of 23 cocainists, 21 chose this method. I know several of these personally, among others an oto-rhinolaryngologist and other scientists, etc. The pursuit of science is not enough to prevent folly. As in the case of morphinism there are instances of husbands perverting their wives to the habit, and mothers their children. In one of the latter cases a morphio-cocainist brought her fourteen-year-old son, within three months, to a daily consumption of 4 gr. of cocaine. But much larger quantities of cocaine are consumed.

I am able to sketch the physical and intellectual life of a cocainist who, like many others, came to me in his misery for help. On account of a facial neuralgia he had frequently taken morphia until a dentist plugged cotton-wool soaked in a 15 per cent solution of cocaine into several carious teeth. From that time onward the need for morphia disappeared. Carious teeth served as receptacles for the cocaine tampons, i.e. places from which the cocaine passed into the blood, and that in abundance. At certain times he pressed these cocaine plugs between the teeth. The greater part of the cocaine passed into the stomach with the saliva. This particular method of application had not existed hitherto but likewise had fatal results. It was introduced in ever-increasing quantities—finally over 1 gr. daily. The unfortunate man's own words were as follows: "With regard to the action of cocaine on my personality, I can honestly declare that the past five years can be counted among the happiest of my life, and I owe this primarily to cocaine. Nothing can refute this plain fact." His letter of twelve pages terminates with these words: "Time is necessary to bring my conception of the world to a point which is founded on the sentence: God is a substance!" The latter phrase impressively shows in an undisguised fashion the whole effect which cocaine exerts on the brain. The individual is so attached to his periods of delight that everything else, even the future, is despised, although the evils which the approaching catastrophe is absolutely certain to bring with it slowly become apparent even to him.

Will-power diminishes, and indecision, lack of a sense of duty, capricious temper, obstinacy, forgetfulness, diffuseness in writing and speech, physical and intellectual instability set in. Conscientiousness is replaced by negligence, truthful people become liars, and the lover of society seeks solitude. One of my patients said he had "lost his amiable smile." The yearning for the narcotic stifles the voice of life and humanity.

The destructive action on the cerebral functions becomes more apparent. The frequent insensibility which often alleviates the misery of the morphinist is completely missing. In contradistinction to the morphinist, the cocainist finds it very difficult to hide his present being behind the mask which society, tradition, and good manners maintain. His internal loss of balance becomes apparent without suppression. Like all narcomaniacs, the cocainist displays a myopia as to his fate, a limitation of his field of vision in the future. He lives only in and for the moment of indulgence of his passion. For him, its slave, it is the best part of the present and the future, even when he is consciously shaken by the force of the toxin. Mental weakness, accompanied by irritability, erroneous conclusions, suspicion, bitterness towards his environment, a false interpretation of things, groundless jealousy, etc., bring about in the individual, now suffering from insomnia, illusions of the senses while fully conscious. Hallucinations of vision, hearing, smell and taste, disturbances in the sexual sphere and the general condition master those who are severely affected. In many cocainomaniacs confusional insanity preceded by general mental disorders, vacancy of mind as in delirium tremens, extreme alarm due to false impressions, set in. A cocainist who had snuffed 3.25 gr. cocaine armed himself for protection against imaginary enemies; another in an attack of acute mania jumped overboard into the water; another broke the furniture and crockery to pieces and attacked a friend.

Abnormal sensations in the peripheral nerves cause the patient to believe there are animals under his skin. The result is frequently self-mutilation, and by a false application of subjective impressions, the mutilation of members of his family, in order to remove the foreign substance from the body. A woman injured herself with needles in order to kill the "cocaine bugs." A man who suffered from twinges and pains in the arms and feet thought he was being forcibly electrocuted. He thought he could see electric wires leading to his body. Attacks of fury and convulsions generally terminate the malady. In the case of a morphinist and cocainist who took of the former 2 gr. and of the latter 8 gr. daily, these attacks were similar to epilepsy, with unconsciousness and no recollection of the fit. In other cases, especially those in which the last dose was excessively increased, spasmodic cramps and convulsive fits may be accompanied by opisthotonus, fever and irregular respiration.

Korsakov's psychosis belongs to one group of mental diseases, cocaine paralysis to another.[23] I have frequently observed, for example
in the case of the cocainist described above, a gradual increase in the
extent of physical disturbances such as paleness, loss of appetite, extreme emaciation, reduction of urinary excretion, weakness of the
sexual functions accompanied by augmented erotic desires, palpitation and irregular activity of the heart, colour-blindness, diplopia, disturbances of speech such as stuttering, paraphasia and an irresistible
impulse to utter the thoughts, etc.[24] Special symptoms can be ascertained in those cocainists who sniff the drug: eczema and swelling of
the nose, especially at its tip, formation of ulcers on the nasal septum
and sometimes perforation of the same, morbid changes of the muscles,
all kinds of disturbances of the sense of smell, and frequently a modification towards mimicry, unmotivated laughing, and a fixed stare.

The end is predetermined. Lucky the cocainist who, shrouded in
the darkness of mental derangement, is not conscious of his fatal and
tragic destiny. A long time before, many of them have a foreboding of
the track along which their passion, owing to the paralysis of their
will-power, is relentlessly forcing them. In this respect they behave in
the same way as the morphinist, with the difference that the devastation in the cerebral functions occasioned by cocaine is more violent
and the inner exclusion of the individual from moral and social life
takes place more rapidly and coarsely.

The infringements of law committed by cocainists are numerous and
various. Illicit traffic in cocaine, smuggling, the illegal supply of cocaine
to cocainists, and its unlawful acquisition by addicts have given occasion
to many punishments. There are also more serious offences: theft, fraud,
forgery, burglary, robbery with violence, committed in order to obtain
cocaine or money or goods for its purchase. Criminal offences against the
person, such as crimes against morality, murder in a state of cocaine
intoxication, etc., have also occupied the courts. Punishment nearly
always follows. Nevertheless we cannot allow that these patients are in
possession of their free will if we admit at the same time that they obeyed
a strong internal constraint, that they were incapable of correctly utilizing new impressions, but that on the contrary these new impressions
combined with reminiscences of the past have confused them. It is of no
importance in this case whether we consider this state as a permanent
disturbance of consciousness or as a transitory morbid state of cerebral

activity. If in such an individual a pronounced disposition to talk and perform actions of a megalomaniacal character can be ascertained, then his free will must be denied if the offences of which he is accused contradict his real personality and the actual situation in which he committed the crime. That is, of course, if the deed was quite foreign to his true character and could be explained only by the circumstances. If this is not the case, the criminal is responsible for his actions, but should be recommended to the mercy of the judge.[25]

The cocainist, like the morphinist, is nearly always aroused too late from his delightful state of euphory and somnolence to painful reality. One of them whom I disillusioned wrote to me: "The first impression your letter gave me was that of a sentence of death. It seemed to me as if you considered my case hopeless and myself lost without the possibility of salvation." The determined man pulled himself together, diminished the dose of cocaine, drank a great amount of wine, took veronal—but his fate fulfilled itself as I predicted.

These unfortunate beings lead a miserable life whose hours are measured by the imperative necessity for a new dose of the drug, and with each such dose the tragedy of life and of death takes a step further towards the inevitable end.

Many seek refuge in the only remedy applicable, immediate withdrawal of the cocaine. The statements made above as to demorphinization apply also to cocaine. The acute reaction of deprivation gives rise to symptoms which when viewed from outside seem less serious than those of morphia. Fewer groans and lamentations are uttered, and the craving for the cocaine is less violent. But the real suffering due to the deprivation in the cells of the cerebral cortex is nevertheless serious and varied enough to cause the patient to fear a stay in a sanatorium. It is a question of a stay of a year or more, not merely a few weeks. But a cure must be effected wherever it is possible. In some exceptional cases only general uneasiness, twitching of the limbs, sickness, perspiration at night, and respiratory disturbances occur. Generally palpitations and weakness of the heart, with collapse sometimes accompanied by unconsciousness, vomiting, and very occasionally diarrhœa set in. States of extreme anguish and hallucinations always occur in this terrible condition. A short time after the withdrawal of the drug, a young woman morphio-cocainist suffered from a maniacal delusion of persecution, and from hallucinations of hearing and smell of a most serious kind. She showed on her arm, for instance, "death spots" (injection scars) which she believed had been made in a mysterious fashion. She imagined she could tell by the odour of her toilet requisites that she was persecuted. She thought she was to be forced to commit suicide, she saw her husband sitting on a tree. In short, she expressed during more than a fortnight all those foolish ideas of which a depraved mind is capable. There were certain days in the meantime when her temper was serene and her occupations those of a normal woman. On the entreaty of the patient and her family she was given another dose of 0.2 gr. cocaine in order to facilitate the withdrawal of the last remainder of morphia, and the old condition returned. The patient made obscene proposals, believed herself persecuted, and this state of sexual excitation, during which she accused her husband of unnatural vices, etc., lasted several days. Gradually her condition improved.

During the period of weaning from the drug psychotherapy may be combined with the general medical treatment. Unfortunately there are no firm scars of recollection and feeling of the experienced pleasurable sensations which led the cocainist to his addiction and finally into the cocaine pool of infamy. A very small percentage of cocainists recover, the rest relapse.

It is difficult to say whether the international efforts to restrict and regulate the traffic and commerce in cocaine will succeed any better than in the case of morphia. For the reasons I have already discussed, I do not think that fundamental changes will take place in the near future. Even if it were attempted to rationalize or suppress its production by force, other sources of supply and methods of distribution would certainly be found. The prevention of all production is absolutely impossible and out of the question, if only because a substance like cocaine which supersedes all other anæsthetics cannot—like morphia—be eliminated.

Nor do I think that its substitute, dextro-psicaine, a synthetic cocaine-isomer which is only half as toxic as the cocaine obtained from coca-leaves, will be of any help, since the supposition that this product, like the other cocaine-isomers, is free from euphoric effects has proved erroneous.

During recent years I have seen among men of science frightful symptoms due to the craving for cocaine. Those who believe they can enter the temple of happiness through this gate of pleasure purchase their momentary delights at the cost of body and soul. They speedily pass through the gate of unhappiness into the night of the abyss.

PHANTASTICA: HALLUCINATING SUBSTANCES

THE PROBLEM OF SENSE-ILLUSIONS

Normal conscious life consists of an interrupted chain of correctly interpreted perceptions, called forth by external or internal excitations. The perceptions and sensations are subjected to the judgment of habit which generally admits of a real or probable relationship between the impression experienced and the real internal or external world. But it is plain, without further explanations, that this judgment, which is based upon the argument from habit, may be false. The attribution of a received sense-perception to a supposed cause is liable to error. Such errors of judgment become most apparent in the case of the interpretation of processes which have no external cause, but have their source in the human organism itself, and take place in the nervous system, especially the sensory nerves and their branches in the brain.

The most exact and exhaustive philosophical and psychological researches into the problem of sense-impressions caused by internal processes have found no way to explain the appearance and the correct or erroneous interpretation of an impression which has its source in a branch of the nerves. Yet this problem is of great consequence in real life. It extends not only to pathology but also into the life of persons whom we cannot call pathological. Are not "internal visions," subjectively considered, real happenings which he who experiences such inward perceptions may regard as true? That is my own view.

When the prophet Ezekiel states that "the heavens were opened and I
saw visions of God, . . . a great cloud, and a fire enfolding itself, and a
brightness was about it, and out of the midst thereof as the colour of
amber, out of the midst of the fire. Also out of the midst thereof came
the likeness of four living creatures . . . Their appearance was like
burning coals of fire, and like the appearance of lamps . . . as for their
rings, they were so high that they were dreadful; and their rings were
full of eyes round about them four," or "above the firmament that was
over their heads was the likeness of a throne, as the appearance of a
sapphire stone; and upon the likeness of the throne was the likeness
as the appearance of a man above upon it," or that he heard "the noise
of their wings like the noise of great waters, . . . as the noise of an
host," we must inquire into the cause of such internal visions and
perceptions, which in other forms also have for thousands of years
been recorded by persons who were vitally healthy, mentally sane and
at the same time fully conscious of themselves. In other words: have
visions and hallucinations a material cause? Yes, in my opinion. The
nature of the cause need not always be the same, but it is always an
excitation localized in the interior of the body. It is present in the
state of ecstasy and inspiration, when the person attains the highest
concentration of his internal forces on sensation and representation,
and his mental activity is at its maximum as well as in the sense-
aberrations of subjects with an abnormal mentality. In cases of the
former kind there is no need for believers, among whom I number
myself, to doubt the divine inspiration.

It is in such an ecstasy, which eliminates the sense-life of the external world where emotion is plastic and real, that Faust, "seeking
with his soul," cries:

> The heavens arch over me—the moon hides her light—the lamp
> disappears! Vapours arise! Red rays flash round my head. A quiver-
> ing whisper blows down from the valult and makes me shudder! I
> feel it, thou hoverest near me, the spirit I implored. Unveil thyself!

Even is we consider this state as a hallucination of vision and
perception, that is to say as a negation of reality, it conveys a real and
plastic life of the soul, like the religious visions of Benvenuto Cellini
when imprisoned in the dungeons of St. Angelo, and other which

have been described in times past on the part of many other individuals, saints and others, the so-called visionaries.

I assume that a material cause originating in the sexual sphere influenced those female visionaries who in the Middle Ages and later achieved notoriety through their singular behaviour, for instance Christine Ebner, who gave rise to much criticism at the end of the thirteenth century. From her fourteenth year onwards she had visions and dreams accompanied by excitation. She felt that she had conceived of the Holy Ghost, gave birth to Jesus, suckled him, and enjoyed his caresses when he grew to manhood. Under conditions unknown to us the human body is able, without the aid of bacteria, to produce substances about which we in our days are only beginning to surmise—substances endowed with the property of producing intermediary states between health and sickness, or even genuine disease, including abscesses and mental disorder.

I have defined disease as the result of the effect of foreign influences.[1] Visionary states are likewise, in my view, generally temporarily limited intermediate and transitory states caused by substances produced in the organism. The action of these substances brings about in the individual subjectively felt realities, which should not be subject to the reproach of fraud or untruthfulness, such as Meister Eckhart, the greatest representative of fourteenth century mysticism, laid to the charge of visionaries:

> If it is said that our Lord from time to time speaks with good people, and that they hear words, such as in some cases: Thou art of the elect, I have chosen thee, and so on, such words must henceforth not be believed.

If, in order to investigate how these internally caused perceptions appear and to which cause we must attribute them—false projection of ideas, unreal happenings or non-existent objects—we limit the problem to what we can actually observe, we are immediately faced with a tangible cause to which psychologists and alienists ignorant of the facts have paid little attention, and which for this reason has not been followed out to its final consequences—I mean the action of chemical substances capable of evoking such transitory states without any perfectly normal mentality who are partly or fully conscious of the action of the drug. Substances of this nature I call Phantastica. They are capable of exercising their chemical power on all the sense, but they influence particularly the visual and auditory sphere as well as the general sensibility. Their study promises one day to be of great profit for the understanding of the mental states above mentioned. Many years ago I indicated the part played by chemical substances of another kind in the appearance of mental disturbances of some duration, and very recently in the case of a gas, carbon monoxide, I pointed out briefly how genuine permanent mental diseases may be produced by a disturbance, as the issue of my own investigations in the sphere of the hallucinants or Phantastica shows.

The problem is as follows. Taking for granted what we know of the Phantastica and of their action as chemical substances on the brain in the form of sensorial illusions, may we go further, and suppose that in those cases where hallucinations and visions transitorily appear in perfectly sane persons they are due to the chemical action of bodies produced for some reason in the human organism itself? We may presume that there is a certain mental predisposition present at the time. We may base our affirmative response on facts. I know of organic products of disintegration which actually cause temporary excitation of certain points of the brain. I know of others which bring about somnolence and sleep and even mental disorders. Even if other causes are brought forward to explain hallucinations, if they are interpreted as the consequence of the excitation of certain central nerves, all these interpretations do not exclude the possibility of the chemical action of certain bodies produced in the organism being the direct cause of the excitation and the indirect cause of the series of consequences.

The importance of the Phantastica or Hallucinatoria extends to the sphere of physiological, semi-physiological and pathological processes. It throws light on the concept of excitation, not easily accessible by science, on which so many strange manifestations of the cerebral functions are founded, by giving it an explanation without which it would be void, an explanation which accounts for the various effects by the chemical action of chemical substances produced in the organism itself. An objection to this point of view should not be found in the rapid appearance and eventual rapid cessation of the phenomena and the restitution of normal sense-perceptions. There are many chemical and especially chemico-catalytic reactions which develop in the same manner. I am convinced that it is the chemical action of organic decomposition-products which causes the hallucinations so frequently met with in febrile diseases, hallucinations which the patient shows in such abundance and such a variety of forms even when he has not completely lost consciousness. If any light is ever to be shed on the almost absolute darkness which envelopes these cerebral processes, then such light will only originate from chemistry, and never from morphological research. Morphology indeed has succeeded hitherto in giving but few explanations of vital processes. It has given no explanation of the extremely delicate action of certain chemical substances on living beings, especially on their nervous system, and will in all probability remain equally sterile in the future.

The point of view here put forward does not pretend to be the only one applicable to know processes of life. Others assume, in my opinion with equal justification, that a religious impulse, for instance, a truly divine emotion which makes the soul vibrate in its most profound depths, may be transmitted as a wave of excitation, and may influence centres which call forth internal impressions, false perceptions, hallucinations, etc. I know from events of everyday life[2] that very violent emotions may under certain favourable conditions give rise to certain changes in the cerebral functions. These emotions are not only such as may be considered as aberrations of the intelligence, fear, anguish, fright, horror, but also the repulsive instincts such as disgust, loathing, abhorrence. The disorders of the brain which these sensations evoke are most various, collapse, delirium, convulsive trembling, troubles of the vascular system, etc. They may even terminate in death through the secondary reactions of vital organs. These consequences certainly appear more frequently than is supposed, but the mechanism to which they are to be traced is extremely difficult to perceive.

It was once thought, in order to explain the incomprehensibly sudden fatal action of prussic acid, that mere contact with the mucous membrane of the mouth, for example, is sufficient to produce a "dynamic effect" similar to the production of light and darkness when an electric current is switched on or turned off. How the poison could be absorbed, conducted to the brain and have time to act so rapidly as to explain the extremely sudden death could not be imagined. This conception has proven to be erroneous since prussic acid, in spite of the great rapidity of its deadly effect, has been traced in the brain. I mention this fact because it throws light on the wide difference between the two theories explaining the appearance of abnormal activities in the brain.

The following pages will also show how Phantastica as miraculous thaumatrugic agents combined with religious and superstitious ideas have been highly esteemed and utilized in past days, and are still so used by some people at the present time. This we can understand when we know their properties, the properties of evoking sense-illusions in a great variety of forms, of giving rise in the human soul as if by magic to apparitions whose brilliant, seductive, perpetually changing aspects produce a rapture which is incessantly renewed and in comparison with which the perceptions of consciousness are but pale shadows. Harmonious vibrations of sounds beyond all human belief are heard, phantasms appear before men's eyes as if they were real, always desired but never attained, offered to them as a gift from almighty God. These properties explain why many of these substances have been and are used for illegal purposes.[3]

ANHALONIUM LEWINII

History of the Plant

"The Teochichimekas (the genuine Chichimekas) know herbs and roots, their properties and their effects. They also know of peyotl. Those who eat peyotl take it instead of wine, as well as the poisonous mushroom nanacatl. They assemble somewhere in the prairie, dance and sing all day and all night. The next day they meet again and weep to excess. With their tears they wash their eyes and clear their brains (i.e. return to reason, see clearly again . . . The plant peyotl, a kind of earth nopal, is white, grows in the northern parts, and produces in those who eat or drink it terrible or ludicrous visions. This inebriety lasts two to three days and then disappears. The Chichimekas eat considerable amounts of the plant. It gives them strength, incites them to battle, alleviates fear, and they feel neither hunger nor thirst. It is even said that they are protected from every kind of danger."

This quotation is taken from Sahagun,[4] the principal Mexican chronicler, who first mentioned peyotl in his works about forty years

after the conquest of Mexico by Fernando Cortez. The naturalist
Hernandez, who lived in the reign of Philip II, and had seen the plant,
but only pointed out as characteristic the striking white silky pappus,[5]
had heard that those who ate its root could predict the attacks of
enemies and their future fortune, or reveal the hiding place of stolen
goods.[6] In more recent religious works it is stated that the Church
attributed diabolic properties to the magic effects of peyotl and urged
the priests to make inquiries about it in the confessional. Hence the
book of Father Nicolas de Leon, *Camino del cielo,* "the Road to
Heaven," contains the following questions for the priest to ask the
penitent: "Are you a fortune-teller? Do you predict future events by
reading omens, explaining dreams, or tracing circles and figures in
water? Do you adorn with flowers places where idols are kept? Do you
know of magic formulas which bring luck to the hunter or make rain
fall? Do you suck the blood of others? Do you go about at night to
invoke the aid of demons? Have you taken peyotl or given it to others
to drink in order to discover secrets or the whereabouts of stolen or
lost property?" Another work[7] contains the following reply of an Indian to a question during confession: "I have believed in dreams, in
magic herbs, in peyotl and in ololiuhqui, in the owl . . . etc."

Until 1886 nothing was known as to the nature and character of
this substance. At this time the plant came into my possession during
my travels in America. Hennings, of the botanical Museum of Berlin,
recognized it as a new species of anhalonium. It received the name
anhalonium lewinii. My first examinations[8] of the plant proved that it
contained alkaloid substances, especially a crystallized alkaloid called
by me anhalonine, which has, like the plant itself, extremely strong
excitant properties capable of provoking muscular cramp in animals.
As a result of experiments nothing was learnt of the processes of excitation in the sensitive and sensorial sphere, but it was proved for the
first time that there was in the family of the cactuses, hitherto regarded as biologically harmless, a species possessing considerable and
general toxic properties.

This discovery and others which followed excited a lively interest
in the application of anhalonium as a narcotic. They gave rise to subsequent researches, of which the chemical and biological investigations proved very valuable, whereas the flood of botanical research
was with a few exceptions unproductive. I myself obtained from the

ripe seeds of my specimens the first plants of *a nhalonium lewinii henn.*, and had them examined by experts.[9] It is botanically related to *anhalonium williamsi* but differs from this morphologically and to a greater extent chemically. *Anhalonium lewinii* contains four alkaloids, among them the vision-producing mescaline, whereas *anhalonium williamsi* contains only one, Pellotine,[10] which is free from such properties. This fact alone should suffice to differentiate the two.[11]

Its Uses

Like the poppy, this anhalonium towers above the rest of known plants on account of the special character of its effects on man. No other plant brings about such marvelous functional modifications of the brain. Whereas the poppy gradually detaches the soul and the body with it from all terrestrial sensations and is capable of leading them gently to the threshold of death and setting them free, a consolation and a blessing for all those who are wearied and tormented by life, anhalonium procures for those who make use of it, by its peculiar ex-citation, pleasures of a special kind. Even if these sensations merely take the form of sensorial phantasms, or of an extreme concentration of the inner life, they are of such a special nature and so superior to reality, so unimaginable, that the victim believes himself transported to a new world of sensibility and intelligence. It is easy to understand why the Indians of old time venerated this plant as a god[12] and looked on it as the vegetable incarnation of a divinity.[13]

The use of the drug has now lasted for hundreds or thousands of years, over rather a limited area, it is true, and will continue to do so in spite of the regulations of Governments (the United States of America has prohibited its use) until the plant, which grows in places remote and difficult of access, may perhaps in days to come be ex-hausted. It is found in the dry plateaus of the north of Mexico in the States of Tamaulipas, San Luis potosí, Queretaro, Jalisco, Aguas Calientes, Zacatecas, Cohahuila, etc. In the north of Cohahuila not far from the railway which now runs through the Eagle Pass along the Rio Grande del norte to Villa Lerdo, there was in 1692 a mission station with the name "El Santo Nombre de Jesus Peyotes," or Pellotes, which still exists as a village. Behind this place rises a chain of hills called Lomerios de Pellotes. The name Peyotes is derived, as the old chronicles state, "de la abundancia en los peyotes." The use of peyotl and the rites which accompanied it were probably know to all the tribes from Arkansas to the valley of Mexico and from the Sierra Madre to the coast, among others from Huicholes, the Tarahumari Indians in the State of Chihuahua, the Indians of Texas, the Mescaleros Apaches, who derive their name from the plant, and the Omaha, Comanches, and Kiowas in the territory of Oklahoma. In every one of their respective idioms the plant has a different name: señi among the Kiowa, wokowi among the Comanches, ho among the Mescaleros, hikori or hikuli in the Terahumari and Huichole tongue. The merchants of the Indian territories call it Mescal (mescal or muscal buttons), the Mexicans on the Rio Grands peyote, peyotl, pellote. These names all indicate the upper part of the plant *anhalonium lewinii*.

This consists of dry lumps, of a grey-brown colour and an irregular circular form, approximately 1.5 cm. high and 4 cm. in diameter. They have rugose protuberances, spirally situated, which are covered with thick tufts of whitish-yellow tomentum, and the summit is crowned by a thick and woolly cushion of a dirty white colour. It is probable that other species of anhalonium with a less powerful or different action passed by the name of peyotl. Those who do not themselves collect the plant buy it.

The plant was considered sacred by the aborigines, and was persecuted as a work of the devil by the missionaries who placed the eating of it on the same level as cannibalism. According to Mooney the ceremony of peyotl-eating among the Kiowa lasts from twelve to twenty-four hours. It starts at 9 or 10 o'clock and lasts sometimes till noon the next day. Nowadays the night from Saturday to Sunday is generally devoted to this purpose, in accordance with the white man's view of the Sunday as a holy day and a day of rest. The worshippers sit in a circle round the interior of the sacred tipi with a fire in the middle. At the beginning of the ceremony the leader prays, and then passes four anhaloniums to each man, who rapidly consumes them. He first removes the layer of hairs, chews the cactus, takes the substance from his mouth, rolls it in his hands, and swallows it. Singing and the noise of drums and rattles accompanies the sacred rite.

An Indian from Omaha who had taken part in a sitting of peyotl-eaters states that baptisms are also celebrated with a concoction made by stewing the plant. The novice is baptized in the name of the Father, the Son, and the Holy Ghost, wherein the anhalonium plays the

part of the last-named. The concoction is drunk. It is also used to
make signs on the forehead of the novice, who at the same time is
fanned with an eagle's wing. This use of anhalonium in religious ceremonies, which can be paralleled in the case of other hallucinating
substances, suffices to convey an idea of the tremendous impression it
exercises on the unconscious sensibility of man. Torn for some hours
from his world of primitive perceptions, material wants and necessities, such an Indian feels himself transported to a world of completely
new sensations. He hears, sees, and feels things which, agreeable as
they are, must of necessity astonish him because they do not in the
least correspond with his ordinary existence and their strangeness must
create the impression of supernatural intervention. In this way anhalonium becomes God, as the patient I have already mentioned stated
that God was incarnated in cocaine.

The Huichol generally eat peyotl only in December or January
during a kind of harvest festival. Starting in September or October
special expeditions are organized for gathering it in the high steppes,
which generally last forty-three days. All those who participate in this
sacred pilgrimage carry a painted tobacco calabash as an emblem of
priesthood. During this time they refrain from consuming salt and
paprika, and from coition. The gathering of the plant in the appointed
place is accompanied by special ceremonies, of which the principal
consists in the repeated shooting of arrows to right and left of the
plant. During the festival the dry anhalonium is grated and mixed
with water, and the resulting thick beverage is handed to the men and
women at regular intervals. Then the hallucinatory phenomena
appear.

Hallucinations due to Peyotl

In the action of peyotl, as in every case of man's reaction to an influence, one factor must be taken into account as an essential element in
the form taken by the reaction: the individuality of the subject. There
are no means of foreseeing this form. It is impossible to lift even a
corner of the veil that shrouds the physiological process in the diversity of the functional modifications of cerebral life subject to the influence of one of these substances. Hallucinations of vision, such as
we shall shortly describe, may be completely absent, and hallucinations of hearing and disorders of the feeling of location in space may

take their place. I consider it important that no single component of the plant, mescaline for instance, represents its total action. The other substances present in the anhalonium which in part may act differently co-operate and exercise an influence on the total result.

Influenced by the quantity imbibed—more than 9 gr. have been taken—the effects appear after one to two hours and may last four or more hours. After an injection of mescaline the effects generally last five to seven hours. They come about in darkness or when the eyes are closed, but may also continue if the subject passes into another room.

It is not always possible to distinguish sharply between the different stages. The first phase, generally accompanied by unimportant physical sensations, consists in a kind of removal from earthly cares and the appearance of a purely internal life which excites astonishment. In the second phase appear images of this exclusively internal life, sense-hallucinations, miracles which affect the individual with such energy and force that they appear real. During the greater part of the time they are accompanied by modifications of the spiritual life which are peculiar in that they are felt as gladness of soul or similar sensations, impossible to be expressed in words and quite foreign to the normal state, but nevertheless full of delight. No disagreeable sensations disturb these hours of dream-life. The troubles which are liable to occur in the sense-illusions of certain mental diseases, sensations of fear or disturbances of action, never appear. The individual is usually in a state of extreme good humour and full of a feeling of intellectual and physical energy; a sense of fatigue rarely occurs, and then, as a rule, only during the latter course of the toxic action.

The sense-illusions are the interesting factor at these stages. Quite ordinary objects appear as marvels. In comparison with the material world which now manifests itself, the ordinary world of everyday life seems pale and dead. Colour-symphonies are perceived. The colours gleam with a delicacy and variety which no human being could possibly produce. The objects bathed in such brilliant colours move and change their tints so rapidly that the consciousness is hardly able to follow. Then after a short time coloured arabesques and figures appear in endless play, dimmed by black shadows or brilliant with radiant light. The shapes which are produced are charming in their variety; geometrical forms of all kinds, spheres and cubes rapidly changing

colour, triangles with yellow dots from which emanate golden or silver strings, radiant tapestries, carpets, filigree lacework in blue or on a
dark background, brilliant red, green, blue, and yellow stripes, square
designs of golden thread-work, stars with a blue, green, or yellow tint
or seeming like reflections of magic crystals, landscapes, and fields
bright with many-coloured precious stones, trees with light-yellow blossoms, and many things besides. As well as these objects persons of
grotesque form may frequently be seen, coloured dwarfs, fabulous creatures, plastic and moving or immobile, as in a picture. At the end of
the psychosis one man saw with his eyes open white and red birds,
and with closed eyes white maidens, angels, the Blessed Virgin, and
Christ in a light blue colour. Another patient saw her own face when
she closed her eyes. An increase of sensibility to variations of light
can be ascertained as in the case of strychnine.[14]

These internal fantastic visions may be accompanied by hallucinations of hearing. These are more rare than the former. Tinkling and
other sounds are heard as from very far away or are perceived as the
singing of a choir or a concert, and are described as wonderfully sweet
and harmonious. Sometimes agreeable odours are perceived or a sensation as if fresh air were being fanned towards the subject; or unusual
states and feelings are experienced. The general sensibility may be
affected, and then the subject has the illusion of being without weight,
of having grown larger, of depersonalization, or of the doubling of his
ego. The body of an epileptic had become so insensible that he did
not know whether he was lying down or where and how he was lying.
The sense of time is diminished or is completely lost.

It is significant that in all these abnormal perceptions due to functional modification in the cerebral life the individual preserves a clear
and active consciousness, and the concentration of thoughts takes
place without any obstacle. The subject is fully informed as to his
state. He exhibits a desire for introspection, asks himself for example
whether all the strange things he experiences are real. But he rejects
this idea, well knowing that he has taken anhalonium. Nevertheless
the same phantasms impose themselves upon him once more. A man
to whom the preparation has been given said to the physician: "I know
I am in my senses and I thank god for having let me see such beautiful
visions. They ought to be shown to jewellers and artists, they might
be inspired by them." This was the man who believed himself to be in

the heavenly kingdom and who had seen among others the Blessed Virgin of Czenstochova.

The most important fact in the whole mechanism of the cerebral cortex is the modification of the mental state, the modification of psychological life, hitherto unknown spiritual experiences compared with which the hallucinations lose in importance. An unprejudiced physician who was placed under the influence of the substance[15] (mescaline), gave the following detailed description of his wonderful experiences:

My ideas of space were very unusual. I could see myself from head to foot as well as the sofa on which I was lying. All else was nothing, absolutely empty space. I was on a solitary island floating in ether. No part of my body was subject to the laws of gravitation. On the other side of the vacuum—the room seemed to be unlimited in space—extremely fantastic figures appeared before my eyes. I was very excited, perspired and shivered, and was kept in a state of ceaseless wonder. I saw endless passages with beautiful pointed arches, delightfully coloured arabesques, grotesque decorations, divine, sublime, and enchanting in their fantastic splendour. These visions changed in waves and billows, were built, destroyed, and appeared again in endless variations first on one plane and then in three dimensions, at last disappearing in infinity. The sofa-island disappeared; I did not feel my physical self; an ever-increasing feeling of dissolution set in. I was seized with passionate curiosity, great things were about to be unveiled before me. I would perceive the essence of all things, the problems of creation would be unravelled. I was dematerialized.

Then the dark room once more. The visions of fantastic architecture again took hold of me, endless passages in Moorish style moving like waves alternated with astonishing pictures of curious figures. A design in the form of a cross was very frequent and present in increasing variety. Incessantly the central lines of the ornament emanated, creeping like serpents or shooting forth like tongues towards the sides, but always in straight lines. Crystals appeared again and again, changing in form and colour and in the rapidity with which they came before my eyes. Then the pictures grew more steady, and slowly two immense cosmic systems were created, divided by a kind of line into an upper and a lower half. Shining with their own light, they appeared in unlimited space. From the interior new rays appeared in more luminescent colours, and gradually becoming perfect, they assumed the form of oblong prisms. At the same time they began to move. The systems approaching each other were attracted and repelled. Their rays were broken into infinitely fine molecules along the middle line. This line was imaginary. This image was produced by the regular collision of the rays against one another. I saw two cosmic systems both equally powerful in appearance and the difference of their structure, and in perpetual combat. Everything that happened in them was in an eternal flux. At the beginning they moved at a giddy speed which gradually changed to a quiet rhythm. I was possessed with a growing feeling of liberation. This is the solution of the mystery, it is on rhythm that the evolution of the world is finally founded. The rhythm became more and more slow and solemn and at the same time more strange and indescribable. The moment drew near when both the polar systems would be able to oscillate together, when their nuclei would combine in a tremendous construction. Then everything would become visible to my eyes. I would experience everything, understand all, no limits would bind my perception. A disagreeable trismus tore me away in this moment from the supreme tension. I gnashed my teeth, my hands perspired, and my eyes burnt with seeing. I experienced a very queer muscular sensation. I could have detached separately every single muscle from my body. I felt great unhappiness and profound discontent. Why had physical sensations torn me from the supremacy of my soaring soul?

However, I had one unshakable conviction: Everything was ruled by rhythm, the ultimate essence of all things is buried in rhythm, rhythm was for me a medium of metaphysical expression. Again the visions appeared, again the two cosmic systems, but at the same time I heard music. The sounds came from infinity, the music of the spheres, slowly rising and falling, and everything followed its rhythm. Dr. B. played music, but it did not harmonize with my pictures and disturbed them. It came again and again, that mighty tension of the soul, that desire of solution, and then each time at the decisive moment the painful cramping of the muscles of the jaw. Crystals in a magic light with shining facets, abstract details of the theory of knowledge appeared behind a misty vaporous veil which he eye sought to pierce in vain. Again forms appeared fighting one another: in concentric circles, from the middle Gothic, from the outside Romanesque forms. With an increasing jubilation and daring the gothic pointed arches penetrated between the Romanesque round arches and crushed them together. And again, shortly before the decision, the gnashing of teeth. I was not to penetrate the mystery. I was standing in the midst of the evolution of the universe, I experienced cosmic life just before its solution. The knowledge was exasperating. I was tired and experienced bodily suffering.

Thus does the character and extent of the action of this marvelous plant present itself. It will easily be understood that, as I have already stated, it will evoke in the brain of an Indian the idea that it is a personification of God. The phenomena to which it gives rise bring the Indian out of his apathy and unconsciously lead him to superior spheres of perception, and he is subjected proportionately to the same impressions as the cultivated European who is even capable of undertaking an analysis of his concomitant state. The physical phenomena which occur in either subject, such as, for example, nausea, a feeling in the breast, heaviness of the feet, muscular spasms in the calves of the leg or the masticatory muscles, are unimportant and without consequences. It is at present not possible to state to what extent the habitual administration of this substance will produce an inner desire to prolong its use, or whether anhalonism, like morphinism, produces a modification of the personality by a degradation of the cerebral functions, as I consider probable.

Thus anhalonium constitutes a large field for research work as to the physiology of the brain, experimental psychology and psychiatry. It is necessary that this work should be carried out, by reason of the richer scientific results we may expect from it than from experiments on animals.

INDIAN HEMP: CANNABIS INDICA

It is recorded that in the year 1378 the Emir Soudoun Sheikouni tried to end the abuse of Indian hemp consumption among the poorer classes by having all plants of this description in Joneima destroyed and imprisoning all the hemp-eaters. He ordered, moreover, that all those who were convicted of eating the plant should have their teeth pulled out, and many were subjected to this punishment. But by 1393 the use of this substance in the Arabian territory had increased.

Four hundred years later the attention of the authorities in Egypt was drawn to the craving for hashish, and on 8th October, 1800, a French general issued the following regulations:

Art. 1. Throughout Egypt the use of a beverage prepared by certain Moslems from hemp (*hashish*), as well as the smoking of the seeds of hemp, is prohibited. Habitual smokers and drinkers of this plant lose their reason and suffer from violent delirium in which they are liable to commit excesses of all kinds.

Art. 2. The preparation of hashish as a beverage is prohibited throughout Egypt. The doors of those cafés and restaurants where it is supplied are to be walled up, and their proprietors imprisoned for three months.

Art. 3. All bales of hashish arriving at the customs shall be confiscated and publicly burnt.

These regulations manifest the spirit of Napoleon, who had left Egypt shortly before this. The measures taken against this substance were the result of direct observation of its action. They were just as successful as were the recent prohibitions of the cultivation of the plant in Egypt. The drug is supplied by smugglers who procure it from Greece. The passion for this substance defies all obstacles, and extends throughout the immense territories of Asia Minor, Asia, and Africa, where it is indulged in by several hundred million people.

The plant in question is *cannabis indica*, Indian hemp, which is not outwardly distinguishable from *cannabis sativa*. In India several preparations are made from it for consumption. In the narghile or water-pipe *ganja*, i.e. the blossoming tops of the non-fecundated female plant, is mostly smoked, as well as *charras*, the resin from this part of the plant. This is obtained by rubbing the tops between the hands, working them with the feet, or rubbing them with a rough cloth. Often a man walks through the field where the plant is cultivated and the resin is then scraped off the leather apron he wears. For preparing the beverage *bhang* the coarsely powdered leaves of female resinous plants are generally used.[16] In other parts of the world the leaves are simply mixed with seeds and filled into the pipe, or the combustion product of the lighted mixture is inhaled by other primitive and unclean methods.

Although the preparations of Indian hemp to be found in commerce are generally of a rather uncertain action, Indian hemp is a very powerful narcotic when employed in its countries of origin. Its use probably dates from about 2,000 years back. Innumerable generations have shared in its consumption, and will probably continue to do so as long as the plant can be obtained growing wild or in cultivation. It has been recently stated[17] that the Assyrians knew of hemp in the seventh or eighth century before Christ and used it as incense. They called it "Qunubu" or "Qunnabu," a term apparently borrowed from an old East-Iranian word "Konaba," the same as the Scythian name *Κάνναβις* (*cannabis*), which latter designation the plant bears at the present day, and as the word "Kanabas" which is derived from the primitive Germanic word "Hanapaz." These words are evidently identical with the Greek term *κοναβος*, i.e. noise, and would seem to originate from the noisy fashion in which the hemp smokers expressed their feelings.[18] This furnishes us with the means of interpreting some statements of the ancient historian Herodotus (486–406 B.C.) He mentions that the Scythians of the Caspian and Aral Seas cultivated a plant whose seeds on combustion produced an intoxicating vapour. The other assumption, that the plant in question is one of the belladonna group, is hardly probable. Diodourus, who lived under Julius and Augustus, also mentions the plant. According to him the women of Thebes prepared a beverage from it which had an effect similar to that of Nepenthes. In the second century Galen expressly points to hemp as a substance in general consumption. He states that at dessert small cakes were passed round which increased thirst, but if taken in excess produced torpor. Toward the year 600 its use extended from India to Mongolia. Ancient Sanscrit writers speak of "Pills of Gaiety," a preparation based on hemp and sugar. In more recent times, especially in the sixteenth century, the reports of its use are more numerous. Garcia ab Horto for example found it very much in vogue in India as a euphoric and hypnotic. Prosper Alpini moreover gives us information about the action of the drug. He relates that on imbibing a preparation of the cheap powdered leaves, the people were intoxicated, and remained for a long time in a state of ecstasy, "accompanied by the visions they desired."

We have learnt quite recently how, thanks to these visions, the drug penetrated into certain regions and how in the thirteenth century and later the "Assassins" (Hashishins, herb-eaters) made use of it to gain novices who served as their docile instruments, fanatical and ready to undertake dangerous political coups and even murder. Through hashish, i.e. by means of hemp, they provoked artificial enthusiasm, ecstasy, inebriety of the senses and at the same time satisfaction of sensual desires. Abbot Arnold of Lübeck wrote in the twelfth century: "Hemp raises them to a state of ecstasy or folly, or intoxicates them. Then sorcerers draw near and exhibit to the sleepers phantasms, pleasures and amusements. They then promise that these delights will become perpetual if the orders given them are executed with the daggers provided."[19]

Those who were influenced in this way committed many evil deeds.[20] These illusions have captured and still in our own days capture men who desire to pass from the misery of actual existence to pleasurable delights within. And how immense are the lands this drug has conquered!

The Extension of Cannabinism in Africa

In Egypt the inhabitants at the present time continue to smoke hashish or to make use of certain preparations adapted to their particular taste. To a great extent this is also the case in North Africa, from Tripoli to Morocco. The drug is used in Tunis, and in the district of Rirha to the east of Biskra the Arabs consume large quantities. They prefer hashish to opium, the action of the former being more rapid and the inebriety of a different kind. The passion for hemp increases towards the east. The whole of Algeria, especially Kabylia, is to-day full of hashish-smokers in spite of the efforts which the French have been making for many years to suppress the evil.

The Moroccans, as a rule, never take alcoholic beverages, but they like *kif*. Preparations from hemp are also called in those parts Shira and Fasuch. The Arabic name Benj is also used. According to the preparations in my possession Shira consists of light brownish, very agreeably smelling, easily pulverized lumps very powerful in their action. The habit of smoking hashish is very popular among the poorer classes. Among the greater part of them, especially among the camel and donkey driver, the necessity for a bout of inebriety from kif appears every few days. The more refined inhabitants of the towns and the people of the country living close to nature rejected the smoking of hemp up to the end of the last century. In out of the way quarters of many towns small shops can be found where kif smokers indulge in their vice. Years ago there were no less than twenty-seven hashish-smoking dens in Wasan where kif was openly supplied to the customers.

The inhabitants of the Rif and the rest of the Atlas, however, constitute the greater number of the consumers of Indian hemp. Old and young indulge therein from the coast of the Atlantic to the Sahara and Cyrenaica. Those who return from the groups of oases in Central Sahara report under strictest secrecy that the men of the Senussi order intoxicate themselves with hashish before preaching their penitential sermons or accomplishing ecstatic ceremonies, as is the custom among these people.[21] The plant grows there at the highest altitudes in sunny and sheltered spots and is frequently cultivated together with tobacco. After the harvest it is dried and cut on boards reserved solely for this purpose. The finely cut hemp is smoked in very small pipes at the end of long and slender stems (*sibsi*). After a few whiffs the *sibsi* is emptied, refilled, and passed to the neighbour, who smokes, fills it again from his own supply, passes it on to his neighbour, and so on till the round is finished.

In Bornu the smoking of hemp is indulged in scarcely or not at all.

On the west coast of Africa the passion for the drug may exist in isolated parts, but is more apparent in the territories where the Congo Negroes live, for instance in Liberia on the banks of the Messurado River, in the grass prairies of Oldfield, on the banks of the Junk River, near Fisherman Lake and Grand Bassa. They smoke the fresh or dried leaves in pipes in which a piece of glowing charcoal is placed. The cultivated hemp plant is called "Diamba." The pipe consists of a calabash, the open stem of which serves as mouth-piece, the bowl of clay being fixed to a hole in the side of the gourd.

On the banks of the lower Ogowe the Ininga smoke hemp, whereas their neighbours the Fan are not addicted to the vice.

Along the coast of Loango hemp is smoked in water-pipes. The leaves and seeds are used, and are according to samples in my possession sold in long thick rolls similar to sausages wrapped in tow. In Angola the different tribes do not smoke hemp in the same manner. Whereas, for instance, the Ngangela smoke but rarely and clandestinely, the Tjivokve have a passionate love for the narghile filled with hemp. Farther south there is a region where the smoking of hemp has become a popular custom. This can be asserted of the Bergdamara in Nama- and Damaraland, of the Ovambo, and to a greater degree of the Hottentots, Bushmen, and Kaffirs. The happiness of Kaffir consists in lying on his back the whole day long and occasionally taking a whiff of hashish, the *dacha*. The Zulu Kaffirs place a handful of the dacha on the ground and some burning manure on top, cover both with earth and dig air-holes on both sides with their fingers into the little heap. Then they lie down one after another and each takes a few whiffs, retaining the smoke in the respiratory organs, a practice which is always succeeded by a violent attack of coughing and expectoration. Instead of these earth pipes, kudu or other horns and calabashes are employed as narghiles. The Bushmen consume the drug in ordinary tobacco pipes. The Heigum, i.e. those who sleep in the bush, smoke hemp they themselves cultivate, which is also called Heigum (*haium*). It brings sleep to those in the bush. The Auin men and women also avidly smoke hemp cultivated by Kaffirs in Oas and Bechuanas in Chansefeld, as well as by white farmers, from whom they procure it by way of exchange. Occasionally they cultivate it themselves in primitive fashion. In the south of central Africa, for instance in Manbunda, Matabele, and Rhodesia in the Zambesi region, hashish is smoked extensively. The Makololo and the Batoko call hemp or the smoking of hemp *muto kwane*. Its use extends further to Mozambique—in Quelimane hemp is called *ssrúma* or *dumo*—and is especially common in the territory of the Congo.

In these parts certain relations appear between the custom of smoking hemp and religious conceptions or national and ritual organizations. It would seem that sects of some kind are founded on its use. There may be found in diverse forms, in particular among the Kassai tribes, a cult of "Riamba." The Baluba, for instance, meet at night for a religious ceremony in order to smoke hemp. The hemp-smokers have formed a sect among some of the Baluba, neighbors of the Bachilange on the banks of the river Lulua. They call themselves "friends." Large parts of the land round their villages are sown with hemp which is hardly sufficient for their wants. The cultivation is carried out on a kind of communistic basic. The cult of Riamba practised by the Baluba was compulsorily introduced by the chief Kalamba-Mukenge. He sought to create a new religion. The ancient fetishes were destroyed and in their place hemp was introduced as a magic and universal means of protection against all injury to life and as a symbol of peace and friendship. The partisans of Kalamba therefore call themselves Bena-

Riamba and greet each other with the word *Moio* (life). They are forbidden to consume palm-wine, but it is their duty to smoke hemp. According to Wissman's description all festivals are celebrated with Riamba banquets, and when smoking the Riamba (a huge calabash more than a yard in diameter, from which everyone takes three or four whiffs) pacts of friends are made and business transactions concluded. The man who commits a misdeed is condemned to smoke a certain number of pipes of hemp under supervision until he loses consciousness. The pipe accompanies the men on voyages and in war. Every evening the people meet in the Kiota or principal square of the village to smoke hemp. The silence of the night is generally interrupted by spastic cough attacks of zealous riamba-smokers. In Luluaburg also hemp-smoking plays an important part, but not to the same extent as in the region of Kalamba.

Hemp-smoking is also greatly in vogue in East Africa, with the exception of the territory between the lakes. It commences to the east of Lake Tanganyika. The Wanyamwesi cultivate the plant everywhere. They smoke the hemp which they themselves produce in narghiles of calabashes, and also snuff hashish. They call the plant "njemu." On the coast of Khutu and Usegua, for instance, it is abundantly cultivated. The consumption of hemp is very considerable in the districts around Lake Victoria, for instance Usukuma, Ututwa, Uganda, Kavirondo, Karagwe, Ukerewe. The Wassinyanga, the Washashi and Néra people cultivate the drug and smoke it to excess, whereas it has penetrated only to a slight extent into some East African territories, for instance the Tanga coast. It is frequently to be met with among the Nyam and in Kordofan, where, although prohibited, it is sold in the marketplaces. In Madagascar hemp is called "vongony."

The Use of Hemp in Asia Minor and Asia

The cultivation of hemp formerly flourished greatly in Turkey, but was prohibited towards the end of the last century, though this did not prevent its clandestine use. A preparation is in use called *Esrar*, i.e. the secret, which is smoked together with tobacco. Hemp in other forms is also chewed. In Syria hemp is cultivated and the resin carefully collected. In Damascus there are many dens where opium and hashish are smoked. Both substances are used in Persia. In this country *Heshish* is obtained by rubbing for hours on end the flowering tops and leaves of the plant on coarse woolen carpets, so that the resinous juice, which is too thick to penetrate into the carpet, is deposited on the surface. It is scraped off with the aid of a knife and rolled into small balls or irregular oblong sticks of a dirty green colour. The carpets used for this purpose are then washed with a small amount of water which is afterwards evaporated in the sun in porcelain plates. In this way an inferior product is obtained. It is said that nux vomica is added to some preparations of hemp. So far back as the beginning of the last century Mehemet Khan punished those who used hemp beverages with death.

The Uzbeks and Tartars are addicted to hemp. The natives of Turkestan prepare hashish for their own use. In the time of the native Khans the sale of hemp was severely punished, but naturally without avail. In Shiva many persons, including the Dervishes, are addicted to the vice, which extend to Afghanistan and Baluchistan. In the Pamirs, amid the ice and snow, Bonvalot met Afghans who were on their way from Kashgar to Kabul over the Badakshan bringing cotton fabrics and hashish.

In some provinces of India, those of the north-west for instance, the cultivation of hemp, and in particular the manufacture of ganja for smoking, is prohibited by law. As a substitute bhang is produced, from which a hashish beverage is prepared. Considerable amounts of hemp preparations are consumed in Hindustan. In Kashmir large quantities of cannabis grow on the banks of the Jhelum and the Vishan, a strip five yards wide being reserved for the cultivation of the plant on each side, and the right of gathering it let out on lease. The leaves are not smoked, but an intoxicating product, Majun, is prepared from them.[22] The inhabitants of Bhutan high up in the Himalayas are passionately addicted to hemp-smoking. Charras is a very important object of commerce in the markets of Khatmandu in Nepal. In Bengal also there are many hemp-smokers. In certain parts merchants allow would-be smokers to take a few whiffs from a large pipe (Hukka) on payment of a fixed charge. The habit is to be met with throughout Eastern Asia, as well as in the north up to the oasis of Shami, where the Chinese Mohammedan tribe of the Taranche are addicted to it, and in the south in Burma and Siam, etc. It is always present, though not always in the same degree, for in some places, although it exists, it is little developed.

The Indian Yogis and their miracles may also be mentioned here. Among other things they have visions, and are capable of passing into trances and cataleptic states. The Yogi Haridās is said to have remained for forty days in a state resembling death, and even to have been buried. We must suppose that in order to obtain this result some kind of narcotic was taken, for instance hemp in the form of Bhang or Ganja; the latter is recommended for this purpose in Sanscrit texts. I think it likely, however, that this action is due to the application of datura or hyoscyamus, whose active principle, scopolamin, is frequently employed in medicine to produce somnolence; and this is confirmed from other sources.

In other parts of the world the employment of Indian hemp as a narcotic agent is unimportant. But it is said that the Chinese coolies in British Guiana are addicted to its use together with that of opium, and that they are supplied with these two substances under the control of the authorities.

The Effects of Indian Hemp

The course and character of the acute effects of hemp depend upon the nature and quantity of the preparation applied, and the individual disposition of the consumer, i.e. his physical and mental state, and so on. According to the general opinion hemp is smoked principally in order to increase the sexual functions or to experience voluptuous sensations in the trance state. This may be true, but it is not possible to quote precise facts as to the positive results obtained in this respect. It is possible that in the beginning some erotic visions intermingle with the dreams of the short and imaginary life into which the smoker of hashish is transported. These visions doubtless make this state desirable. Perhaps sexual potency is increased at the outset, but it nevertheless diminishes during the subsequent addiction to the drug, as in the case of opium-smoking.

After the first impressions of anxiety and restlessness hemp produces in most cases a feeling of happiness, the result of a sense of physical well-being and internal content. This state may manifest itself as an exhibition of gaiety in which the smokers behave in a very childish and stupid manner. At the same time peculiar convulsive laughter may be observed, the consequence no doubt of hallucination or bizarre illusion. After this attack of laughter one or other of the

smokers starts weeping, giving his passion as the reason. Faintness may mark the beginning of this latter state.

There are other occasional consumers of hashish whose mental life is said to take the form of a wonderful dream, all the nuances of which are determined by the individual's environment and intellectual standard. In the most favourable case his impression is that all the thoughts which pass through his brain are lightened by the sun and that every one of his movements is a source of joy. Such men are not happy in the same way as the epicure or the starving man who satisfies his hunger, or the voluptuary who gratifies his desires, but like one who hears good news, a miser counting his treasures, a gambler favored with luck, an ambitious man intoxicated with success. At the same time a certain state of confusion may be present in which all kinds of far-away thoughts, of which he seeks an explanation in vain, attack the individual. Confused schemes which hitherto seemed unrealizable become simple before his very eyes and approach realization. The bonds of time and space are broken.

Hallucinations, especially of sight, hearing, and general sensibility, frequently accompany the effects described. The last-named are usually of a disagreeable character. The senses become finer and more subtle. For instance, the impression made by noises is quite out of proportion to the real sounds emitted. If a person in this state talks or laughs his ear is affected as if by the thunder of cannon; a murmur gives the impression of a waterfall. Fireworks, rockets, and many-coloured stars seem to fly from the head. This state may be temporarily interrupted by the appearance of disagreeable sensations. Mortal fear makes the individual shiver and at the same time he is attacked by violent electric shocks. He feels as if he were put in irons or his brain devoured by fire. Occasionally, however, harmonious enchanting music is heard. A delicious joy and a feeling of intense well-being reappear. The illusion of being raised into the air may occur, and the subject seems to be clinging to a tree or experiencing the terrible sensation of expecting from moment to moment a fall into the abyss. This latter impression of danger has sometimes also been produced by some of the medicinally applied hemp preparations. The effects of the toxin may last several hours. Alterations of taste have also been observed, generally after the termination of the principal effects. Dishes served in a restaurant to a person under the final influences of the drug were of an unheard of savouriness. A deep sleep concludes the whole process.

There are also other varieties of the acute stage of intoxication. Some African hemp-smokers, for example, after a few whiffs become quite incapable of responsibility. Naturally it is quite impossible to obtain any enlightenment as to their internal sensations. Other hemp-smokers, after smoking a great deal, remain sitting with a fixed stare and a hanging under-lip, and a continuous nervous shivering shakes their bodies. Livingstone relates of the hemp-smokers of the Zambesi that after the first violent attack of coughing has passed and the excessive salivation is in progress a torrent of senseless words or phrases is uttered, such as "The green grass grows," or "The cattle are in the pasture." Nobody pays any attention to this flood of eloquence. Other smokers pass into a state of inebriety and ecstasy, leap and bound about until faintness and exhaustion throw them down. Europeans who smoke hemp frequently exhibit an abnormal desire for movement. They run about the room and a host of wild nonsensical ideas is let loose in them, which are impulsively expressed often with the accompaniment of bursts of laughter. Under the influence of an impulse of this kind a person who had taken hemp was compelled to crawl on his hands and feet. Although he was quite conscious of his actions he had no desire to do anything else. Finally there are individuals who after imbibing large quantities of hemp preparations manifest no nervous excitation, but a profound torpor or even a state of coma. Riff pirates smoking kif may be seen squatting apathetically in a corner meditating in silence, indifferent to the outer world. Some burst occasionally into shrill laughter, while others only grin placidly to themselves. One imagines himself the son-in-law of the chief, another thinks himself at sea and makes desperate swimming movements in order not to sink with his plank-bed. A third commands a troop of imaginary slaves to perform senseless and impossible deeds, and a fourth explains to everyone who will listen that he is really a great magician and tomorrow is going to hurl into the sea the rock-bound castles of the Spaniards.

The habitual smoking of Indian hemp, chronic cannabinism, after a certain time modifies the faculties. It changes the character in a humanly and socially unpleasant direction. Moroccans who were in the service of Europeans proved serviceable and reliable until they smoked kif. In users of Indian hemp the same craving for the drug appears under the same conditions as for opium and cocaine. Hemp-smokers indulge their passion daily or every three to five days. Ebn Beithar at the end of the twelfth century declares that hashish inebriates in doses of 4 to 8 gr., that larger doses give rise to delirium and insanity, whereas habitual consumption produces mental weakness or raving madness. This is the case. In such persons the intellectual faculties are weakened, and, according to the old Arab's saying, bad habits and spiritual debasement are produced so that they sink below the level of mankind. The whole populations of villages round the basin of the Kassai are morally and physically ruined by hemp, and it is reported of the Wanyamwesi that a great part of them have become half imbecile through its abuse.

For some time information has been forthcoming from the lunatic asylums in India and Egypt as to the frequency and modifications of mental diseases due to hemp. The important role which it plays in Bengal in the appearance of these disorders is indicated by the fact that of 232 cases of mental diseases 76 were caused by hemp. Of these latter only 34 were cured. It is said that generally speaking the sudden and rapid cure of such diseases is the only diagnostic sign of insanity due to hemp. In my experience this is only valid for a small percentage of very slight cases. In the lunatic asylum in Cairo, out of 248 inmates, 60 men and 4 or 5 women owed their mental state to hashish. These patients, like the occasional eaters and smokers of the drug, may be divided into several groups.

The first group exhibits a state of general euphory and excitation with visual hallucinations and illusions sometimes extending to deliria which are less violent, less aggressive, and more easily to be influenced than alcoholic delirium. The symptoms of ataxia are not present. A cure may be accomplished in one day. Individuals in a state of excitation may be considered as irresponsible.

The second group is characterized by a state of acute mania. The sense-illusions are terrible and are succeeded by maniacal delusions of persecution, sometimes also by a state of violent fury. The patient is agitated, garrulous, a prey to morbid illusions, and suffers from insomnia. Such cases last several months and are not always curable.

The third and very numerous group comprises mentally weakened persons who pass into a maniacal state after every excess of hashish. During their stay in the hospital they appear calm. Their talkativeness alone discloses their mental state. They are easily satisfied, lazy, without energy, indifferent to the future, without interest for their relatives. Their only desire is to be well fed and to get tobacco. The slightest provocation, however, evokes a state of violent excitation. After dismissal from the hospital they soon fall once more into the state of mania. They are extremely agitated, insult their friends, swear and easily become violent. They deny that they use hashish, immediately after they have praised its wonderful properties. This state of mania is in many cases chronic and ends in incurable dementia. These individuals seldom commit crimes.

Besides bronchitis and dysentery caused by the irritants contained in the hashish-smoke, this passion gives rise to general physical deterioration. The smokers of hashish may be recognized from a distance by their pale faces, hollow cheeks, and insecure gait. The offspring of inveterate hemp-smokers are liable to be of inferior quality if conception took place during inebriety. Among the Riff pirates scrofulous children are known as "Uld l'Kif," i.e. son of kif. What can be considered as true of alcohol in this respect is also valid for hemp, a substance of quite a different kind. The spermatozoa are subjected to the injurious effects of the active principles of hashish and are in this state conveyed to the ovule. It seems to me probable that the craving for hemp can be inherited.

If, as in India, hemp is consumed with the addition of *stramonium datura,* then the resulting maniacal state and dementia are greatly facilitated.

Everything I have stated about cannabinism tends to prove that the substance in question is a Phantasticum of a kind which, besides giving rise to sensorial illusions that are not always agreeable and to individually occurring feelings of intense well-being, is apt to develop extremely brutal effects leading to mental diseases. This impression of well-being is seated in the soul and cannot therefore be localized in the brain. Attention must be drawn to the differences between these mental diseases and those produced by cocaine. In both cases the active agent is a chemical substance. The process of the reaction is just as obscure as with other substances of a similar nature. Is the action in question an irritation? If this be assumed we must endeavor to find the reason for the difference in the qualities of the irritation which evoke such extremes in functional alterations of the activity of the brain. Even if this were known another problem arises. Why is the repeated action of these two substances so different and why does it extend to different parts of the brain? If in all these problems a chemical action or an action founded on chemical affinity were assumed, as I have already stated, we would gain more insight into the causality of the action of these substances. Certain components of hemp must be regarded as having a specific relationship to certain points of the brain which results in local modifications having the consequences described. These apparent effect are quite dissimilar for instance to those of *anhalonium lewinii* which calls forth utterly different, and we might almost say nobler, alterations of the functions or the state of certain groups of ganglia.

The abuse of hashish cannot be prevented in spite of severe regulations. Although in the French part of Africa the smoking of hashish is prohibited, and although it is also mentioned in the new law relating to the restriction of the traffic in opium, cocaine, etc., it is smoked in spite of the difficulty of obtaining the drug. If its use is prohibited in public places, the passion is nevertheless indulged clandestinely. Public scandal is avoided, but the craving itself is all the more protected because it is hardly or not at all to be observed. If the cultivation of Indian hemp organized in Germany in 1917 for medicinal purposes should furnish hashish suitable for ordinary consumption, a new source of toxicomania would be established.

FLY-AGARIC: AGARICUS MUSCARIUS

The passionate desire which consciously or unconsciously leads man to flee from the monotony of everyday life, to allow his soul to lead a purely internal life even if it be only for a few short moments, has made him instinctively discover strange substances. He has done so even where nature has been most niggardly in producing them and where the products seem very far from possessing the properties which would enable him to satisfy this desire. In North-East Asia, in the territory of Siberia, through which the Obi, Yenisei, and Lena flow, bounded on the north by the icy Siberian Sea and on the east by the Bering Sea, the Samoyeds, Ostyaks, Tungus, Yakuts, Yukagirs, Chukches, Koryaks, and Kamchadales in ancient times discovered in the *agaricus muscarius*, the *muchamor* of the Russians, properties which supply them for hours together with what for them is happiness. This is the well-known poisonous mushroom, which has been the object of intense chemical research. Nevertheless, further scientific efforts are necessary in order to identify its active elements, particularly those which give rise to hallucinations. One thing is certain, the substance which caused me to place this mushroom among the group of the Phantastica is not muscarine.

Character of Agaric Inebriety

The effects of the fungus have long been known. The attempt has been made to establish a relationship between them and the accounts according to which the Norwegians or giants of old, called Berserkers, were at times seized by peculiar attacks of fury and savageness. It was assumed that these attacks were due to the consumption of agaric which was taken for this purpose by all the peoples of the North as far as Iceland. This, however, is mere surmise. If it were really the case, then the use of the fungus by the peoples above mentioned must be considered as a relic of its former very extensive employment. It is only since the end of the eighteenth century that precise reports have been forthcoming, especially as to the great demand for the plant. In some parts of the country it cannot indeed be found in quantities sufficient to satisfy the need. This is, for example, the case in the territory inhabited by the Koryaks, and in the Taigonos Peninsula it does not grow at all. From Kamchatka, where it abounds, it is conveyed from merchant to merchant right round the Gulf of Penshina. Formerly the Koryaks paid for the merchandise with reindeer. In winter they frequently exchange an animal for a single mushroom.

In order to obtain the desired effects one large mushroom or two or three small ones dried in the open air or in smoke are sufficient for one day. The smaller agarics with a large amount of white warts are, as the inhabitants of Kamchatka state (in my opinions correctly), more powerful in their action than the pale red and less spotted specimens. Cold or warm extracts of the agaric in milk or water are also frequently consumed together with the juice of *vaccinium uliginosum*, the bog-wortleberry, or the juice of the French willow, *epilobium angustifolium*. The inhabitants of Kamchatka are said to prepare a beverage from the latter plant alone. The Koryaks and the Chukches have been observed to take out small round boxes made of birch fiber or leather which contained small pieces of dried fly-agaric. From time to time they placed one in their mouth and retained it there without swallowing it. Among the Koryaks the drug seems to be used in the following manner: the women chew the dried agaric, and roll the masticated substance in their hands into small sausages, which are then swallowed by the man.

Among the exceedingly numerous problems offered by the fly-agaric not the least important is that the Koryaks, Kamchadales, etc., discovered that the urine of a person intoxicated by agaric also possesses intoxicating properties. Who taught them that the active principle of the mushroom is not destroyed in the organism but is completely excreted in the urine, which then has the same effect on the brain as the agaric itself? As soon as the Koryak notices his inebriety decreasing, he drinks his own urine, if he has no more agarics, or in order to economize. The Koryak women pass a tin receptacle reserved for this purpose to the intoxicated person into which the urine is passed in the presence of all. The urine, frequently still warm, is drunk by the person awakening from sleep and after a few minutes exercises its influence. In this way the action may be renewed several times. If there should be any of the urine left over, it is preserved for a short time to be used on the next occasion. Even during a journey on the reindeer-sledge, when the half-drunk Koryak leaves the camp, he collects his urine in the receptacle which he always carries with him. The urine of another person inebriated by agaric acts in the same way, but, it would seem, only once. A traveller passed near the yurta of a Koryak and wanted an agaric for his domestic. The Koryak, however, was drunk, and passed urine with which the domestic obtained a more prolonged state of inebriety than the Koryak himself had reached. When the latter attempted to make the substance act for a third time, utilizing the urine of the person he had accommodated, failure resulted. It is unlikely that the active principle can be found in the urine in quantities large enough to be effective after having passed through four or five persons. It is not always for reasons of economy or poverty that the urine is employed. It is stated that the Shamans of the Yugakirs and Tungus always imbibe an agaric urine of this kind before consuming the actual mushroom.

The physical and mental condition of the individual has a considerable influence on the modifications of the cerebral functions caused by the agaric. There are not only differences between one individual and another, but also, according to the circumstances, in the same person. The same man may be at one time very susceptible to a single mushroom and at another hardly affected at all by several. On the whole, the effects are very similar. Generally they begin to be experienced in the first hour after consumption, but sometimes not before two hours. In some cases twitching and trembling of the limbs together with subsultus tendinum can be observed. As a rule consciousness is maintained at the commencement and even a slight numbness does not hinder the individual from feeling light on his feet and from still retaining his will-power for a short time. In this state he is in the best of humours and experiences a feeling of internal joy and contentment of spirit. Then hallucinations and illusions set in. He speaks with persons who are not present, but whom he sees with the eyes of his soul. He tells them with delight of the large fortune he possesses, of the wonderful things he sees, and how happy he is. He may also be interrogated by the persons present, and is frequently able to answer quite reasonably, but always in connection with the phantasms which in his state of intoxication appear to be real. He sits there, quite calm, without rage or fury, pale, with a glassy stare, as if dead to his environment. In this state independent actions dictated by free will are possible. A Koryak woman, for instance, was found sitting in a tent in a state of inebriety due to agaric, incessantly beating a drum and quietly moaning.

In 1776 Krasheninnikov described persons who in the absurd manner of very feverish patients became, according to their temperament, extremely sad or excessively jolly. Some jump about, dance and sing, others cry and are prey to "astonishing fright." Illusions of a particular kind accompany these sometimes different forms of inebriety. Through his enlarge pupils the individual sees all objects in a monstrous size and remarks upon this. A small hole seems to be an enormous abyss, and a spoonful of water a lake. This deceptive perception is apt to influence his actions. If a small obstacle is placed in his way, as is frequently done by the Koryaks for a joke, he stops, examines it, and finally jumps over it with a large bound. On the basis of his illusions, the conclusion which he arrives at is very reasonable. Therefore the two points of the brain from which the illusion, the macropsia, the magnified vision on one hand and the reasonable thought on the other, originate, must be different, but the method of connection between them must be the normal legitimate bond of sense-perception and the judgment of reason. The voluntary impulse which leads to the action, in this case to the jump, originates from logical thought, and is transmitted to the muscles in a natural way. I presume that the point of the brain influenced and causing the visual illusions is different from that from which the visual hallucinations are started.

Taken in greater quantities the mushroom evokes all kinds of illusory perceptions. An inebriated person declared that he stood on the edge of hell and the agaric ordered him to fall on his knees and confess his sins. This he did amidst the laughter of his friends. This religious aspect of the effects of the Phantasticum is not unusual. An extremely violent initial excitation also frequently occurs. It may be observed in agaric-eaters gradually to increase and to become a veritable attack of raving madness. A man in this state wanted to rip open his abdomen because the agaric ordered him to do so. In this case, as in the preceding, it was hallucinations of hearing which caused or almost caused these actions.

In other cases the motor excitations dominate at the beginning. The eyes take on a savage expression, the face is red and bloated, the hands tremble violently, and the individual seizes a drum of reindeer leather and dances or rushes about the tent to the noise of the instrument until he sinks down in fatigue and falls asleep. In the latter state, which lasts half an hour to an hour, he sees fantastic and agreeable sights which make him happy. Awakened from sleep the individual staggers about until a new crisis with the same course sets in. This may be repeated several times, an act of violence being in this state quite possible.

Occasional by-effects are vomiting, salivation, and diarrhœa. For easily comprehensible reasons hardly any observations of the harmful consequences of the consumption of the drug have been forthcoming. It must be assumed that in the course of time the incessantly renewed material attack on the brain must bring about a numbing of its functions, which after all is difficult to ascertain on account of the low intellectual standard of the tribes in question. Nevertheless, it is stated that even within these limits of mental inferiority a lessening of the faculties has been observed, sometimes amounting to debility. It must be of no small degree to make an impression under these conditions.

On account of the dangers which this substance possesses for the individual the means of procuring it have been surrounded with difficulties. It is prohibited, for instance, to sell fly-agaric to Koryaks. In spite of this the fungus reaches them, for here, as in other countries, trade laughs at all restrictions and at the dangers connected with an infringement of the law.

SOLANACEÆ

The energy of the noxious solanaceæ of the groups of *atropeœ* and *hyoscyameœ* becomes manifest when their active elements affect the brain, in a peculiar form which is similar or even identical for all representatives of these two species, but quite different to all other solanaceæ. This uniformity of action is the result of the concordance or close relationship in the chemical structure of the active elements. They contain the alkaloids atropine or scopolamine or closely related chemical bodies. These substances, and also some derivatives of the group of solaneœ, for instance *solanum incanum L.* in North-West Africa, have the property of calling forth disorders of the functions of the brain which become apparent in the form of a peculiar excitation followed by a state of depression. This constitutes a very characteristic element of their action and has played an important role in the history of mankind. I have pointed out their great importance elsewhere.[23]

We find these plants associated with incomprehensible acts on the part of the fanatics, raging with the flames of frenzy and fury and persecuting not only witches and sorcerers but also mankind as a whole. Garbed in the cowl, the judge's robe, and the physician's gown, superstitious folly instituted diabolical proceedings in a trial of the devil and hurled victims into the flames or drowned them in blood. Magic ointments or witches' philtres procured for some reason and applied with or without intention produced effects which the subjects themselves believed in, even stating that they had intercourse with evil spirits, had been on the Brocken and danced at the Sabbat with their lovers, or caused damage to others by witchcraft. The mental disorder caused by substances of this kind, for instance datura, has even instigated some persons to accuse themselves before a tribunal. The peculiar hallucinations evoked by the drug had been so powerfully transmitted from the subconscious mind to consciousness that mentally uncultivated persons, nourished in their absurd superstitions by the Church, believed them to be reality.

These substances taken in suitable doses may give rise to a state of dementia lasting for hours and even days. I am certain that it has frequently been employed for purely criminal purposes in order to pass off certain persons as mad and thus accomplish private or political designs. I have met with many cases of this kind in the history of mankind and by means of toxicological analysis proved their real significance.[24]

Many other more repugnant things have been accomplished with these substances. They have served to intoxicate girls and seduce them to immoral acts. This may be done without the victim becoming unconscious; she tolerates the criminal with open eyes but blinded soul, and even, as a result of augmented sexual excitation, complies with his wishes.

Besides other disagreeable symptoms these solanaceæ and their active elements, especially atropine and scopolamine, give rise to hallucinations and illusions of sight, hearing, and taste, which differ, however, from those produced by the other Phantastica. They are not of an agreeable but on the contrary of a terrifying and distressful kind. It is doubtful whether when smoking or eating such substances a state of such supreme internal well-being is obtained which is to be considered as the principal inducement to their habitual use. It has not been possible to obtain a precise statement on this point from the relatively small number of persons who make use of solanaceæ. Cases if poisoning by one or other of these plants do not afford any enlightenment in their respect, and only allow of suppositions as to how the coarse functional disturbances in the brain are felt. The opinion that henbane, the Arabic *benj*, is the nepenthes of Homer is quite erroneous. An elementary knowledge of the effects of henbane suffices to refute this hypothesis.

Henbane (Hyoscyamus niger)

In the first century of our era it was known in Rome that the hyoscyamus comprised numerous species, and that the black variety caused insanity. Such knowledge was already at that time very old. For this plant had already served in ancient Greece as a poison, and as a means to simulate dementia and to evoke prophecies. A primary accidental intoxication must have impressed those present with the fact that the person lost his reason, that his eyes shone and the pupils were enlarged, that he made senseless speeches, became aggressive, had sense-illusions which he took for interior visions, and then fell into a state of somnolence with complete insensibility similar to sleep. From this knowledge to the use of the substance as an anodyne or a sorcerer's potion is only a step. The Middle Ages show us this transposition in practice. The wise Bishop Albertus Magnus, regarded in his days in the thirteenth century as a sorcerer, stated that the properties of henbane played a part in the conjuration of demons by necromancers. The ancient names of the plant, *pythonion* and *apollinaris*, are attributed to the gifts of prophecy obtained by its ingestion.

Recent reports on the impressions of patients who were treated with scopolamine, the active principle of henbane, supply more information. They experience a feeling of pressure in the head as if a heavy body rested on it. At the same time an invisible force seems to close their eyelids. Sight becomes vague and all objects seem to be stretched lengthwise. All kinds of visual hallucinations are produced while the eyes are open. For instance, a black circle on a silver background or a green circle on a golden background appears. The eyes then close and sleep sets in. The senses of taste and smell are also frequently affected. When sleeping the individual is surrounded by fantastic apparitions.

Hyoscyamus Muticus (Hyoscyamus Albus)

The properties described above are very marked in the species of henbane called by the Arabs *sekaran* or *ssakarân*, i.e. the inebriating. It flourishes throughout Egypt, and according to the accounts given by my friend Schweinfurth, very plentifully in the oasis of Shargeh and in the Sinai Peninsula. In the latter the Bedouins, Towara, and others smoke the dry, felt-like leaves and become deliriously drunk.

An application of the same kind of *hyoscyamus muticus* (*hyoscyamus insanus Stocks*) is frequently met with in Baluchistan and the Punjab, where it is called *kohi-bhang* and *kohi-bung*. The inhabitants smoke it in small quantities like Indian hemp.

Thornapple (Daturas Stramonium)

"In the years 37 and 38 Antony set out on an expedition against the Parthians, who opposed an almost invulnerable barrier in the East against the domination of the Romans. Like many others before and after him, not only did he meet with no success, but he was humiliated nearly every day by this warlike people. The retreat of the troops was a very sad one. Provisions were lacking. The army was forced to fall back upon unknown roots and herbs for food, which they first had to test as to their quality. In this way they found a herb that killed after producing insanity. 'He who consumed a little forgot all that he had done and recognized nothing.' He did nothing but turn over every stone he found in his path with the greatest gravity, as though it were a difficult task. There was a field where the soldiers did nothing else."[25]

Judging by these symptoms I consider this plant to be datura or hyoscyamus, more probably the former. Although the similarity of the mode of action of the plants of the group of solanaceæ is very great, there are nevertheless gradations in the symptoms of intoxication which render it possible to determine a particular species with a certain degree of accuracy. The senseless activities and occupation caused by a datura-intoxication are characteristic of this plant. In addition to this the loss of memory corresponding to the period of the intoxication must be taken into account. This has been known for centuries, and has given rise to many crimes. Towards the end of the seventeenth century extensive poisoning by means of the plant took place, which gave rise to the following precise description:

If only a small quantity of the plant is given to a person his mind is depraved and deluded to such a degree that anything can be done in his presence without fear of his remembering it on the following day. This distraction, mental disorder, and madness of his mind lasts for twenty-four hours. During this time you may take his keys from his pocket or open his chests and cupboards before his very eyes. You can do what you like with him, he notices nothing, understands nothing, and knows nothing about it on the next day.

By means of this drug one can do as one pleases with women and obtain anything from them. That is why I believe that there is no more noxious plant in the world, and none whereby such evil things can be accomplished in a natural manner.

Domestics ate a plate of lentils in which by mistake thornapple seeds were contained. They became quite mad. The lace-maker exhibited an unusual zeal and fussiness, threw the weaving-cone to and fro and entangled everything. The chambermaid entered the room and cried at the top of her voice: "Look! All the devils of hell are coming!" A servant carried all the wood into the secret chamber under the pretext that he had to distill liquor. Another hit two hatchets together and said he was chopping wood. Another crept about on the ground, and dug up and scratched the earth and the grass with his mouth like a hog with its snout. Another imagined he was a wheelwright and wanted to pierce and bore holes in all the wood. He then seized a large piece of wood in which a large hole had been burnt, held this hole to his mouth, made swallowing motions and exclaimed: "Now I am almost properly drunk. Oh, this drink tastes good indeed!" This good man intoxicated himself in his imagination with a piece of dry wood and an empty hole. Another went into the smithy and cried for help to catch the fish which he imagined to be there in enormous numbers. This insane herb has evoked all kind of senseless illusions among others. It allotted different tasks to various tradesmen which were carried out without payment and produced farcical results. The next day nobody remembered his ridiculous doings and could not be persuaded to believe that he had acted in this manner.

In our own days men have been seen to follow the most extravagant impulses under the influence of datura, for instance to dance or to climb incessantly. A tailor who had come under the influence of belladonna and datura exhibited the usual dilatation of the pupils as well as severe convulsions. After these symptoms had disappeared he sat upright in his bed after the manner of tailors and made motions as if he were hard at work, threading the needle, etc. In this state he neither heard nor saw what happened around him. This state of unconsciousness lasted for fifteen hours.

More serious effects, however, have been produced by religious fanatics, clairvoyants, miracle-workers, magicians, priests, and imposters in men who in the course of religious ceremonies inhaled the smoke of the burning plant or were forced to imbibe the substance as a beverage. The *herbe aux sorciers, herbe au diable* (magic or devil's herb) served to evoke fantastic hallucinations, illusions, and deceptions. In demonology this plant has played a more important role than the playman ever suspected.

Sense-illusions accompanied by troubles of the motor organs, disorders of the perceptive faculties and orientation necessarily also occur if the leaves or other parts of the plant are smoked habitually for pleasure. This can be ascertained in East Africa among the aborigines and the Arabs. They smoke *datura stramonium* and *datura fastuosa L. (datura alba Nees)*. The latter is called *mnará* and *mnarábu*; datura stramonium passes among the Arabs and Swahili under the name of *muranha*.

In India there are also areas where datura is used, for instance in Bengal. Enthusiastic devotees smoke *cannabis indica* or *ganjah* with two or three datura seeds or a certain quantity of the leaves. In order to reinforce or modify the action of alcoholic beverages on the brain, seeds are crushed into the liquor, which is then strained and mixed with palm-wine. This is practised, for instance, in the province of Madras. In Bombay the fumes of the roasted seeds are brought in contact with an alcoholic beverage for one night. It is certain that the active elements of the plant evaporate and are apt to be absorbed by the alcohol. It is stated that in Japan the leaves are smoked together with tobacco by those addicted to this vice.

It can be gathered from the preceding pages that the effects of datura with their singular illusions and strange disorders of consciousness are known in three continents. But this lant is also not unknown in America. In Darien and in the Choco territory the inhabitants cause children to drink a decoction of the seeds of *datura sanguinea Ruiz et Pav*. During the resulting mental confusion they are compelled to walk. Gradually the initial excitation is succeeded by a state of depression and at the same time a failure of motility occurs. As it is a common belief that the gift of discovering gold is combined with a visionary state, the earth is dug up where the child falls down, and as there is a large quantity of gold in the soil, it is frequently discovered in that place.

Many other Phantastica are said to bestow a like gift of divination. This belief is as ancient as the idea that sense-illusions sharpen the wits and intelligence. The conquerors of Mexico found besides *anhalonium lewinii* a species of datura, *datura meteloides D. C.*, or *ololiuhqui*[26] in use. The latter when imbibed gave the individual the power of discovering stolen objects. The effects of a plant of this kind were at that time excellently described as follows: "*Aiunt multa ante oculos observari phantasmata, multiplices imagines ac monstrificas rerum figuras, detegique ferum si quidpiam rei familiaris subreptum sit*" (They declare that they are able under its influence to see many fantastic apparitions, multiplying and changing images, and wonderful forms, and also to detect a thief).

This datura, *datura quercifolia R. et P. (Brugmansia bicolour Pers)*, and perhaps also *datura arborea L.* and *datura sanguinea H.B.K.* were and still are in our days employed as inebriating substances by the Indians, as well as by the South American tribes which use coca. Tschudi himself observed the effects of *datura sanguinea*, the herb of the graves, *bovœhero* or *yerba de huaca*, and *yerba de Guacas*. The Indian who had drunk the beverage, *Tonga*, prepared from the capsule of the seeds, passed into a profound lethargy. He sat there with convulsively closed mouth and stared at the earth with an empty gaze. After a quarter of an hour his eyes began to roll, he foamed at the mouth, and his whole body was shaken with convulsions. After these symptoms ceased he fell asleep for several hours. In the evening he was found surrounded by a circle of very attentive hearers to whom he narrated how he had communicated with the spirits of his ancestors. From this the name of herb of graves is derived. The Indian priests of old took datura when they desired to enter into communication with their gods or to attain a state of prophetic inspiration. This led to thornapple being identified with the sacerdotal plant of the Oracle of Delphi. However, judging by the symptoms I consider this supposition as unfounded from a toxicological point of view. In Delphi sulphuretted hydrogen containing gases gushed out of a crevice in the earth and acted on the Pythia seated on the tripod.

It is reported that the Red Indians of the Great Salt Lake, the Utahs, and also the Pimas and Maricopas smoke the leaves of *datura stramonium* together with those of *arctostaphylos glauca*, or chew them without an admixture.

The use of plants containing tropeins is frequently rendered impossible by the fact that all the tropeins give rise to serious cardiac symptoms which endanger the functions of the heart and because a habituation to tropeins takes place only to a very slight degree. The brain, however, for a considerable time endures the state of excitation to which it is subjected.

Datura arborea

The field of action of datura arborea is the same as that of the solanaceæ I have already described. It is employed by the South American tribes of the upper reaches of the Amazon as well as farther to the north. The Jibáros call the plant and the beverage they prepare from it *maikoa*, the Canelos Indians *guantuc (huantuc)*. This datura is a shrub found in a wild state in the forests of Ecuador and the subtropical mountainous regions. The Indians, who also cultivate the plant, use it to prepare an inebriating beverage taken in order to obtain revelations from the spirits during intoxication. According to Karsten's observations the bark is scraped off and pressed in calabashes until approximately 200 gr. of the juice are obtained. This is one dose. It is either imbibed at home or in the especially built "Rancho of Dreams." The Indian spends three days in this abode. He is allowed to consume only one roasted unripe banana per day, but as much tobacco-juice and extract of datura as he likes. Among the Jibáros on the Rio Upano or Santiago, when the boys attain manhood, they drink *maikoa* on the festival celebrated on this occasion. Badly behaved boys are made to drink *maikoa* while fasting. This is considered a radical cure. Magicians drink it in order to cure diseases and also to bewitch enemies while in the state of inebriety. Before emptying the cup they chant an incantation. Warriors drink it before a campaign, to learn whether they are in danger, are to live long, etc., and others make use of the drug to procure advice from the spirits or internal visions.

The effects begin with a pronounced impulse to move. Those especially who are not yet used to the toxin strike about them with weapons, sticks, etc. This state of raving madness, similar to that produced by belladonna, may become so violent that the insane person has to be bound by his own followers. In this state he speaks incoherently and suffers sense-illusions of the kind already described. During the festival of puberty the Jibáros hold the boy who has taken *maikoa* from behind until the violent excitation is succeeded by the second period, that of narcosis, into which all the drinkers pass. During the latter visions occur of beautiful plantations, wonderful animals, large pots of beer, and other things which make the heart of the Jibáro rejoice.

In this way knowledge of the action of the tropeins extracted from the solanaceæ and their use establishes a connection between that distant world and ours. The application of this knowledge permits an influence on the soul and the production of momentary states of mental alienation. These states force the individual so far from the path of his ordinary thoughts that it is easily understood how these intellectually uncivilized people attribute their visions to a supernatural and religious origin.

Duboisia hopwoodii

The fifth continent, Australia, also possesses a member of the solanaceæ, *duboisia hopwoodii*, which is used as a narcotic. It only occurs in Central Australia. It is found in great numbers near the border of South Australia between latitude 23° and 24° south and at longitude 138° east, and also approximately 50 miles to the west and east of this district. In the form of bushes its growth extends from the Barcoo River and the Darling River (Queensland) to the border of West Australia. It is not found in Tasmania or Victoria. In all the parts where it is found the plant is assiduously collected. Large expeditions are undertaken for this purpose. The natives make use of it in exchange for other goods. They collect the tops and leaves in August when the plant blossoms and hang them up to dry. They also dry the material under a layer of fine sand, powder it, and keep it in skins or small crescent-shaped satchels.

The plant and the drug prepared from it is named *pituri* (pitchery, petgery, bedgery). The latter represents a lumpy, brown mass, consisting of the powdered leaves of the pituri with its petioles, nerves, and stalks. The blacks of the Wilson River, Herbert River, Cooper and Eyre Creek, and especially the Mallutha tribe, make use of the drug. It is both chewed and smoked. When chewing it a quid is formed which is passed from mouth to mouth. The last chewer sticks it behind the ear of the first. The pituri-chewer masticates the substance and sticks it behind his ear, whence it is taken from time to time, to be finally swallowed. The quid is said to be also prepared with charcoal and employed in the usual manner. The leaves of duboisia are smoked. They are moistened, some alkaline charcoal is added, and they are then rolled into the form of a cigar. This pituri cigar is also chewed and the saliva swallowed.[27]

We are here once more confronted with the remarkable practice of adding alkaline substances to stimulating or narcotic remedies which has frequently been mentioned in this book. This is done in the case of the chewing of coca and betel, and also in that of tobacco. Peoples of all kinds have instinctively found the most suitable means of setting free the active elements of the plant and enabling them to pass into the organism. In pituri an extremely active alkaloid is liberated which is nothing else but scopolamine (hyoscine), also present in thornapple, datura. It is the active principle of the series of solanaceæ with which we have to deal. One tenth of a milligramme often suffices to give rise to serious intoxications. The Australian natives highly value pituri, which violently irritates the mucous membrane of the nose, eyes, and mouth, as a tonic on their long journeys across the desert. Its primary action even on animals is highly exciting, and those who employ it utilize it also in order to obtain courage before battle. They are aware of the extreme toxicity of the product and even use it to poison the large emu.

The case of a man who, in order to break himself of the alcohol habit, for nine months took scopolamine in increasing doses from 0.0005 to 0.002 gr. per day, gives an idea how pituri exercises its effect in larger quantities. He exhibited mental disorders with hallucinations particularly of sight and crazy illusions which are among the typical effects of the tropeins and scopoleins, including belladonna, scopolia, and duboisia. Under the influence of the toxin he lost the sense of locality and did not recognize his habitual surroundings. He talked unreasonably and his memory was weakened. He was cured in several days. In small doses such as are consumed by the eaters and smokers of pituri scopolamine gives rise to hallucinations and illusions, similar to the effects of datura, with the same limitation of consciousness which seems to be so agreeable and detaches the individual from time and space.

BANISTERIA CAAPI

In North-West Amazonia, from the Orinoco over the Rio Negro to the Cordilleras, near the cataracts of the Orinoco, on the borders of the Rio Uaupés, Rio Içana, Rio Meta, Rio Sipapo, Rio Caquetá, on the upper reaches of the Putumayo, and Rio Napo, in the enormous territory which extends over parts of Columbia, Ecuador, Peru, and Brazil, various tribes—in addition to alcoholic beverages and tobacco, and also coca, which is in common use—make use of numerous hardly known plants, especially of *banisteria caapi*, as a Phantasticum. Among others the Guahibo and Tukano tribes (for instance the Correguáje, Táma, Zaparo, Uaupé, Yekuaná, Baré, Baniva, Mandavaka, Tariana, Cioni, Jibáros, Colourados, Cayapas) employ the plant.

The banisteria is a liana of the family of *malpighiaceœ* which occurs in the virgin forests of Ecuador and is also cultivated by the Indians. In Ecuador it is called *aya huasca* in the Quichua language, by the Jibáros *natema*, by the Colorados *nepe*, by the Cayapas *pinde*, and by the Yekuaná *kahi*; the beverage prepared from the plant passes under the same name. Sometimes it is also applied together with other plants, among others perhaps with the liana *hœmadictyon amazonicum*. If the latter is added to the beverage the character of the effects are different, because this plant, which belongs to the species *echites*, is extremely toxic. It is known that, for instance, *hœmadictyon suberectum* (*echites venenosa*) is very toxic and the *echites masculata* secretes a stupifying milky juice. The Indians probably add tobacco-water also to the beverage.

It seems certain that *banisteria*, generally used by itself, evokes mental disorders similar to the effects of datura. In order to obtain these effects, as may be gathered from the excellent observations of Karsten, a piece of the lower part of the liana is cut off, cleaned, and reduced to small lumps. The triturated substance is boiled in water, from two to twenty-four hours, in order to reduce the initial quantity to a small volume according to the activity desired. The latter, however, depends not only on the concentration of the liquid but also on the quantity imbibed and the degree of repletion of the stomach. If the stomach and small intestines are empty the passage of the drug into the lymph-tracts takes place much more rapidly and with greater force. These conditions are realized when caapi is consumed in the usual manner, because certain doses of the substance give rise to vomiting, which is desirable and to a certain degree necessary, as a preparation for the final action on the brain. This vomiting takes place in regular intervals after every new quantity of approximately one litre has been imbibed. In this manner the way is prepared for the absorption of further doses of the narcotic.

Ordinary people take a beverage prepared in a different way from that of the sorcerers, who, in order to discover the causes of and to cure diseases or to bewitch their enemies, add to the already extremely bitter banisteria liquid in the course of ritualistic ceremonies the wood and the leaves of another liania called *jahi*. They are thus transported into a state of ecstasy. This magic plant *jahi*, *yahe*, or *yaje*, is probably identical with the hœmadictyon mentioned above. At any rate it seems to act in the same way as banisteria.

During the boiling of the plant and when drinking the prepared beverage a drum is generally beaten. The Jibáros drink this beverage during a special festival, the Natema feast. This lasts for a week. Men, women, and half-grown children, all who wish to "dream," meet on this occasion. Before passing the cup to the drinkers the dispenser of the beverage murmurs a magic formula. There are many other occasions for Natema drinking, not during a public festival, but at home, and many make use of it habitually. Widows, for example, drink it before choosing a new spouse. It is generally imbibed when a person desires to pass into a state of trance, during which the future and the best possible course of his actions is revealed to him.

Usually the effects of the inebriating beverage are as follows: After it has exercised its action on the stomach in the form of vomiting and has reached the brain in sufficient quantities the drinker is seized with vertigo. He staggers, leans on a stick as long as he can hold himself, and then falls down in a narcosis full of sense-illusions. As a rule, as is the case with all substances of this kind, the narcosis is preceded by a more or less marked state of excitation, during which the subject is very agitated, dances, screams, etc. It is doubtful whether this state is accompanied by convulsions.

The characteristics which make the Indian love the *aya-huasca* beverage are, in addition to the visionary dreams, the pictures bearing on his personal happiness which he sees "in his mind's eye"; beasts in which demons are incarnated or other peculiar (sometimes agreeable) phantoms. Perhaps also sexual impressions are experienced. It seems as if mainly illusions and visions are produced in the mind of the toxicomaniac.

Travellers have occasionally tried banisteria on themselves. Koch-Grünberg, for instance, drank two small calabashes of the magic liquor. After a short time he experienced, especially when he emerged into darkness, a peculiar scintillation in crude colours before his eyes. When writing, shadows like red flames passed over the paper. The dose was insufficient to enable him to experience the sensations produced in the Indians by this Phantasticum. Nevertheless, the incomplete symptoms here described suffice to prove that banisteria gives rise to visual hallucinations like those evoked by *anhalonium lewinii* in a perfect form. After having drunk the beverage another traveller saw beautiful landscapes, towns, towers, and parks, and even wild animals against which he defended himself. This was succeeded by a feeling of sleep. A third case of experimental self-application resulted in the seeing of brilliant circles of light, many-coloured butterflies, and the feeling of a duplication of the personality; such grave physical symptoms, according to the description,[28] that their consistency must be doubted from a medical point of view. The symptoms in question are the following: a very accentuated contracture of the lower jaw-bone muscles and on the other hand chattering of the teeth, as well as a "complete" suppression of the pulse and respiration which occurred while the individual remained fully conscious and continued to think and act in a way calculated to overcome the "poisoning" which had seized him.

The use of this Phantasticum is intimately associated with religious ideas similar to those I have described in the preceding pages in connection with other toxic substances. This association may be accounted for by the fact that the sense-illusions evoked by the drug are taken for actual occurrences by the intoxicated subject. It is a state of the soul which tears him away from the realities of everyday life and makes him acquainted with new, incomprehensible and agreeable things. This spiritual state has become indispensable to the drug-taker and will always remain so.

GELSEMIUM SEMPERVIRENS

The substances described above terminate the series of those drugs which man has most frequently employed in order to satisfy the imperative desire to modify his mental state in an agreeable manner. It is probably that one day other substances will accidentally be discovered which are capable of acting in the same way on the brain. Thus during a severe attack of rheumatism a man took a large quantity of an alcoholic tincture of *gelsemium sempervirens*, a plant which is liable to act on the brain and the medulla oblongata. Noticing an appreciable result he continued to take it, and finally became a slave to the drug. He gradually augmented the quantity, and reached 30 gr. of the tincture in one dose. Slowly he became pale, agitated, and discontented. He wasted away. Hallucination set in, and his state grew worse until disorders of the intelligence appeared. As he continued to increase the doses he fell into idiocy and died in a state of mental confusion.

THE LOCO HERBS

In accordance with a generally acknowledged law, substances with the property of evoking a particular state of well-being at the same time give rise to the imperative necessity of frequently renewing the application of the substance in question. This law also applied to animals, as I have proved by personal experiments with morphia on pigeons. In this respect singular observations have been made in America and Australia of certain plants of the family of papillionaceæ, which have hitherto been neglected from the chemical standpoint.

Horses, oxen, and sheep which have for some time eaten *Astragalus mollissimus Torr.*, in the prairies of Texas, New Mexico, Dakota, Colorado, Montana, etc., exhibit a state of mental excitation and also become the victims of illusions, which cause the animal, for instance, to jump with an enormous expenditure of energy over a small object seen on the ground.[29] If an arm is suddenly lifted before their eyes the intoxicated animals fall down as if paralyzed with fright. They turn round in circles or do other similar things. In horses other sense-illusions are also produced. The animals behave in such a manner that we must conclude that a special state of mental disorder is present similar to the state of man under the influence of alcohol or other substances. This state lasts for months. During this time the animals refuse to take any other kind of food and greedily seek to procure their old fodder, like the morphinist his morphia. This phase of excitation is succeeded by physical decay to which the animals succumb. This is the cause of great losses in cattle breeding.

Swainsonia galegifolia, R. Br., acts in the same way. The intoxicated animals, called in Australia indigo-eaters, keep aloof from the rest of the herd, exhibit disorders of the brain, troubles of vision, etc. They refuse to eat grass and only take this toxic herb. In this case also grave and deadly complications set in.

Oxytropis lamberti produces hallucinations and other states of excitation in horses and oxen.

Of the *Aragullus* those which occur as shrubs have a very pronounced action, for instance, *Aragallus spicatus*, Rydb. (white loco weed), *Aragallus besseyi*, Rydb., A. *cagopus*. It is enough for a horse or a sheep to consume on a single occasion a large quantity of this shrub to render it an incurable slave to the passion as long as the plant is accessible. Indeed, one such animal may induce a whole flock to eat *Aragallus*. Younger animals especially become subject to this craving: the older ones more rarely. If *Aragallus*-eaters are kept in confinement they are cured of the loco-disease. The course of this is as follows: the animals at first manifest an increase of vitality and then gradually general apathy. They stagger like drunkards, and may be seen for days on end standing torpidly in the same place from where it is difficult to move them.

Certain effects of our common broon, *Sarothamnus scoparius*, are known which remind one of those loco. The peculiar short-tailed sheep of the heaths of North Germany, especially the Lüneburger Heide (*Heidschnucken*), have a great preference for it. For this reason it is frequently planted on the heath and the sheep are slowly driven through these plantations, for too much is very injurious. The plant acts on the heart like red foxglove. Some animals, the "drunkards," devour it ravenously and fall into a state of excitation succeeded by complete unconsciousness. In this state they are said to fall an easy prey to foxes or flocks of crows.

INEBRIANTIA

ALCOHOL

Remarks on Acute Intoxication

Acute and chronic alcoholism are as old as alcoholic beverages them-selves. Their explanation must be sought in the particular properties of these liquors and in the dispositions of mankind.

Every person, man, woman, and child, savage native of a distant island or inhabitant of a civilized country, knows what acute intoxica-tion is like. It is described with all its distressing consequences in the world's oldest chronicle, the Bible. Artists have depicted it according to their diverse conceptions in representations of the altered activity of the brain reflected in the physiognomy and the behaviour of the drunkard. Poets and authors have described to the world the effect of alcohol in verse and prose, approvingly and disapprovingly according to their point of view. Humour, irony, and earnest reflection are con-tained in these works which exhibit pure unbiased reality or are de-voted to the exposition from a moral or ethical point of view of the consequences of alcohol abuse. There is a Greek inscription on a tomb more than two thousand years old which a poet composed in the form of an epitaph on the defunct who succumbed to the combined action of alcohol and cold during acute alcoholism.

> Ξεῖνε, Συράκοσιός τοι ἀνὴρ το δ' ἐφίεται Ὄρθων
> Χειμεριας μεθυων μηδαμὰ νυκτος ἴοις.
> Καὶ γὰρ ἐγὼ τοιουτον ἔχω πότμον· αντὶ πολησς
> Πατρὶδος ὀθνείαν κεῖμαι ἐφερράμενος.

> *Wanderer, hear the warning of Orthon of Syracuse.*
> *Never travel at night and in winter when drunk!*

For such, you see, was my unhappy destiny; not at home,
But here I lie, covered with alien soil.

Why is it that alcohol has been and is still the subject of such diversity of opinion? The reason must be sought in the exceptional position which it occupies among the stimulating and narcotic substances, both as a producer of intense or light forms of inebriation and in respect to the effects which are called forth if it is used habitually in large quantities. In addition to this we must mention the ease with which it can be procured, its universal application, and, what is of supreme importance, the numerous possibilities of obtaining it from vegetable substances which in a suitable form are distributed over the whole world. On this earth there has been more than one Noah to make use of grapes in the production of an alcoholic beverage, wine, and to teach others the method. Many others drew their conclusions from accidental observations and became inventors of other fermented liquors.

There was probably never a time or a country in the world where alcoholic beverages were not used on special occasions or even habitually with the same aim and in most cases with the same result, viz. to tear the soul away from everyday life and direct it into another sphere where it is not confined within the walls of plain and customary monotony, or burdened with disagreeable and sad impressions, but on the contrary attains gaiety, temporary happiness, and even forgetfulness. This has always impelled man to the use of alcoholic beverages which are indeed highly suited to produce this result, provided that they reach a fit organism in favourable doses.

This was not only always the case, but it will be so in future as long as man and liquor are on this earth. And if in thousands of years some cosmic catastrophe establishes a new order of things, the new man of the future will once more learn to prepare and delight in alcoholic beverages. He also will undergo the same experience with this intoxicant which countless generations have had before him. He will learn that the desired effects may be accompanied by others of a disagreeable nature which are unpleasant in the experience and objectively repugnant. For this reason the helots were forced to become drunk and in this state were led into the dining-halls to show the young Spartans how debasing drunkenness is.

The disagreeable secondary effects are produced according to the same laws which govern the effects of every medicine or toxin. They are nevertheless influenced in their form by individual factors. At all times, for instance, there have been men who after a fit of alcoholic excess were affected with vomiting, as is shown in an ancient picture of 1,500 years before our era[1], i.e. dating from the new Egyptian empire, which represents a woman in the act of vomiting. They also experienced troubles of the motor organs, mental disorders, loss of consciousness, and other grave effects. The consequences of an occasional excess, which is nothing else but an acute intoxication, influence the organism for a relatively sort period of time if no specially aggravating circumstances are present. However, they excite our aversion, because they reveal to us the fact that the individual has, voluntarily or involuntarily, infringed the laws of society.

The force of the reactions with respect to the apparent obnoxiousness has at all times depended on the sensitiveness of the observer. This latter has extremely wide limits, from the most tolerant indulgence to the most severe condemnation. It is just this different estimation which explains the various verdicts arrived at when the intoxicated person has committed an act against the law. Medical men must judge the mental state of the offender at the moment of his culpable act as in every other case where doubts arise as to the free will of the delinquent. On the other hand, if no infringement of the law takes place, and only an alcoholic excess is present, then, in my view this is a purely private concern of the individual. It is the business of other persons just as little as the voluntary state of cocainism or morphinism, or the state of caffeine inebriety produced by drinking large quantities of strong coffee, or excessive gambling, etc. Everybody has the right to do himself harm, and under normal circumstances this right may not be taken from him so long as he is not liable to military service. To some extent acute alcoholic intoxication, although easily mended, nevertheless causes damage to the organism. In this way it was frequently regarded in ancient times, and Plato is to a certain degree right when he makes Eryximachos say in the *Symposium*: "It seems to me indeed quite clear that inebriety is very injurious to man." Here we must take into consideration chronic alcoholism, the state of drunkenness.

Chronic Alcoholism

By chronic alcoholism I understand the state of a person who is led by a strong inclination or craving to taking daily or at regular intervals a dose, which may be very large, of a concentrated alcoholic beverage, so that it gives rise in him to functional disorder of the brain, of which he is himself conscious and which others perceive, and finally to organic modifications. This acquired state corresponds to our conception of inebriation, and a person in this state is an alcoholic. If we transfer this definition to real life, it will be seen that it is applicable to some only of those individuals who take alcohol. Drunkards are sick and therefore unhappy persons. They are also a calamity for their country if they are numerous, particularly because drunkenness renders impossible that regular work upon which a country's prosperity is founded.

The alcoholic is unhappy because he is usually aware that he is a prisoner in the iron embrace of his passion. The action of alcohol diminishes or annihilates will-power. From this point of view, and here only, does alcohol resemble morphia. Essentially there are great differences between the two substances and the impulses to which they give rise. The craving for alcohol is not so violent as that for morphia. No racking pains of the nerves, no state of extreme misery occurs such as takes place after the action of morphia on the brain has ceased. Consequently there is no necessity to supply the brian with a new dose. No internal constraint compels the drinker, like the morphinist, to increase the doses administered. When a cure is undertaken in a clinic I have frequently observed that the former does not suffer so much as the latter. It has not been proved with certainty whether or not a withdrawal cure causes delirium.

Even animals may have the taste for alcoholic beverages to such a degree that when the opportunity arises they make use of them with a certain display of intelligence. The horse of a wine merchant was discovered lying in the cellar amidst a heap of broken bottles, striking with its hoofs against the wine barrels. On being lifted up it fell down again. It was completely drunk. For some time its master had noticed that the horse had attacks of vertigo and fell frequently. The animal had been fed to strengthen it after overwork with oats soaked in wine. A lazy servant, instead of mixing the oats with wine, had administered the latter from the bottle. One night the intelligent animal had got loose, opened the latch of the cellar with its teeth, ravaged among the wine and devastated the cellar.

During my experiments I saw a hedgehog which had been presented with a saucer of warm, very sweet brandy drink it at intervals without leaving a drop. Some hours later, exactly as in the case of a human being who had taken too much, the typical symptoms of "seediness" set in.

Alcoholism and Heredity

Alcoholism is a calamity for mankind in yet another respect. Not only does the individual, who is of comparatively little consequence to the activity of the universe, suffer, but his descendants engendered during the state of drunkenness may also be degenerate. This will be understood in respect to alcohol better than in the case of other poisons which intoxicate the organism habitually or *ex professo*. All bodies endowed with poisonous forces with the opportunity to act under these circumstances may influence the spermatozoa or ova and exercise a chemically noxious effect on their functions. The scientific mechanism of the phenomenon is well known as regards alcohol. It belongs to the group of substances which, like chloroform, ether, benzene, carbon sulphide, etc., are capable of dissolving the fatty matter (lecithin, etc.) contained in the organic complex. The possibility of such action is also present in the case of the sperma and the ovum. Both of them may be deteriorated in their functions. That is to say the acute chemical modification to which they are subjected may leave an impression which, transferred to the living being to which they give birth, communicates a morbid disposition, generally in the form of disorders of the nervous system. The known forms of alcohol in all the organic troubles which they evoke act in the same way, but with different degrees of energy.

This can be proved experimentally in fertilized eggs. If different alcohols are injected in an appropriate manner into the interior, conclusions may be drawn as to the relative toxicity of the various alcohols by observing the greater or smaller number of eggs which are hatched and produce normal chickens, the number which are not hatched at all, and the number of those which give rise to freaks (see Table 3).

TABLE 3. ALCOHOL AND DEFORMITY

NUMBER OF EGGS	INJECTION	PROPORTION FOR 100 EMBRYOS		
		NORMAL	NOT DEVELOPED	MONSTERS
24	Water	75	16.66	8.34
63	Ethylalcohol	53.96	11.11	34.93
63	Methylalcohol	23.08	11.11	65.09
24	Propylalcohol	0	12.5	87.5
12	Amylalcohol	0	58.33	41.63

There are three kinds of defects due to alcohol which are liable to appear in the offspring:

(1) The inclination to alcohol.
(2) Mental diseases.
(3) Criminality.

Numerous experiences prove that this is the case. They also prove that alcoholic degeneration may spare the members of the first or second generation, or at least that it does not become apparent among them. With respect to the first and second class of the degenerative influences of alcohol the following table, founded on positive observations, shows clearly alcoholic deterioration.

Of 600 drunkards, the parents and nearest relations were alcoholic or affected with mental diseases in the proportions shown in Table 4.

Other inquiries made at the Bicêtre Hospital in Paris as to the influence of alcohol on the production of degenerate, idiotic, epileptic, and mentally and morally enfeebled children show the sinister role which alcoholism plays in this connection. Table 5 shows the results obtained in an inquiry into the parentage of 1,000 such abnormal children.

The influence of parental alcoholism on the criminal propensities of the offspring has been proved in the case of a family very interesting from a toxicological point of view.

Ada Jucke, born in 1740, lived till after 1800. She was a drunkard, a thief, and a vagabond. In 1874 six of her descendants were in prison. Eight hundred and thirty-four persons were identified as her direct descendants, and the conditions of living were ascertained with accuracy in the case of 709 of these (see Table 6).

TABLE 4. ALCOHOLIC DEGENERATION AND HEREDITY

	DRUNKARDS	MENTALLY AFFECTED
Father	168	3
Mother	9	3
Father and Mother	12	-
Father and Brothers	7	-
Father and Sisters	2	-
Father and Grandfathers	7	-
Mother and Grandmothers	-	1
Uncles	-	6
Aunts	-	4
Grandfathers	12	-
Grandmothers and Grandfathers	2	1
Brothers	16	6
Sisters	-	7
Cousins	-	7
Other relatives	26	-
TOTAL	**265**	**38**

= 40.4%

TABLE 5. THE EFFECTS OF ALCOHOL ON CHILDREN OF ALCOHOLICS

Number of Children	1,000
Alcoholism of father	471
Alcoholism of mother	84
Alcoholism of father and mother	65
TOTAL	**620= 62%**
Cause of malady not ascertainable	171
Parents not alcoholic	209
TOTAL	**1,000**

TABLE 6. DESCENDANTS OF ADA JUCKE	
Illegitimate children	106
Prostitutes	181
Beggars	142
Workhouse Inmates	64
Criminals (7 murderers)	76

The criminals spent 116 years in prison and for 734 years they were sustained by public charity. In the fifth generation nearly all the women were prostitutes and the men criminals.

The primary cause of the injuries to which the brain is subjected is that the alcohol reaches the latter and is retained for some time on account of the frequently renewed application of the drug. At the beginning of the last century, for instance, in the cerebral cavities of a drunkard who was dissected immediately after death, a clear liquid was found which tasted and smelt of gin. The amount of alcohol concealed in the brain after alcoholic excesses has frequently been ascertained in our own days. In one of these individuals 3.4 c.c. of alcohol were found, and in another 1.04 cc. In a third with 720 gr. of brain 3.06 c.c. were ascertained. To my own knowledge the higher alcohols, especially amylic alcohol and the oils combined therewith, attach themselves for a longer period and more powerfully to the brain.

Alcohol gives rise to the preceding symptoms of a general kind. If we turn to particular cases it will be seen that the effects directly or indirectly called forth by the abuse of alcohol are so numerous that few poisons are capable of evoking them in such variety. Only those which react, like carbon monoxide, carbon sulphide, lead, etc., and are endowed with powerful chemical energy can be compared to it in this respect. Primary disorders which pass into the nervous system and into important organs combine with secondary disturbances which depend on the former and follow their own course after they have been initiated.

This is not the place to study in detail the organic troubles caused by alcoholism. They can easily be followed from the general outlines I have given above. Many volumes might be filled with descriptions of the symptoms of alcoholism. They would commence with scenes out of the Bible, and the experience of several thousand years would follow. From whatever epoch these descriptions are taken they will always be similar to each other and will always remain true.

> Thence the pale complexion, the trembling of the nerves of the wine-soaked body . . . the bloatedness of the skin . . . the insensibility and numbness of the nerves, or on the other hand the twitching of the whole body. What shall I say of the inclination of these people to faintness? What of their disorders of seeing and hearing?

These were the words of a Roman nineteen hundred years ago. After the lapse of an equally long period it will still be true that there is hardly an organ or an organic function which is not disturbed in some way or other in episodic, relapsing, impulsive, and habitual drunkards. It is not possible to predict which of these troubles will be produced in a particular case or how they will be produced. "Individual chance," as I may call it, creates extremely various phenomena. But the past also teaches us that the injurious consequences of alcohol will never cease and that man will rather submit to them than renounce it. At the beginning of the first century of our era Martial satirically depicted this in a poem which will always remain true and typical, and which may also be applied to other evils of the same kind.

> Phryx, the worthy drinker, was blind
> In one eye, and the other was running.
> To him said Heras, the doctor: Avoid wine!
> If you continue like this you will see nothing.
> Phryx smilingly answered: Good-bye to thee, my eye!
> And on the spot he had many glasses mixed.
> Do you want to know the end?
> Phryx drank wine and his eye poison.

It seems unnecessary to describe in detail the moral consequences of alcohol in the drunkard. His behaviour towards himself when he is under the influence of alcohol and his conduct towards his family and society, even if he does not violate any laws, leaves much to be desired in respect to moral sense and duty. The higher qualities of the soul suffer first, then the lower ones. The final result of this modification of the character depends upon the individual temperament. "The choleric person is more inclined to fits of passion, the sanguine has a greater tendency to an intense frame of mind, the melancholic person becomes more sombre, and the phlegmatic weaker and more indolent." The complaint which in Egyptian times an anxious father made to his son who drank is still true:[2]

> *I am told you leave your books . . .*
> *You stray from road to road;*
> *The smell of beer . . .*
> *The beer drives away the people (from you)*
> *It is the ruin of your soul (?)*
> *You are like a broken rudder on a boat*
> *Which obeys in no direction;*
> *You are like a temple without a god,*
> *You are like a house without bread.*

Individual Toxic Disturbances in Alcoholism

The drunkard is always violently oppressed by the burden of alcoholism, and it is of little importance whether and to what degree he is conscious of it. The physically organic injuries depend upon the average amount of alcoholic beverages taken habitually, their concentration and individual resistance. It is therefore useless to try to determine the quantity of alcohol which stamps a person as a drunkard. It is also not possible to ascertain the quantity of lead a workman must absorb during his daily work in order to suffer from grave saturnine poisoning. The same is true with respect to the mercury poisoning contracted in dangerous trades. The gravity of the injurious consequences of alcohol depends largely on the degree of resistance of the individual on account of the mysterious role played by adaptation. That is the reason why in some persons physical or mental troubles appear very rapidly and in others after a much longer period. The regulating functions of which the organism disposes may for years do a great deal to help to maintain the faculty of work in the individual. The prolonged resistance to alcohol of these particularly refractory subjects is said to be promoted by the sleep following the drinking of alcohol. Sleep has been considered as a period of recreation for the organism during which time combustion and elimination take place. I regard this theory as of little interest. On the contrary there are a considerable number of individuals in whom the habit of drinking causes extremely rapid and violent disorders of a physical and mental kind. Among them are women, children, and also persons of superior intellect, especially those with artistic gifts.

Besides the ordinary disturbances of the circulatory system, liver, heart, and kidneys, there is in certain individuals a particularly marked disposition to the evil effects of alcohol, and it appears in the evolution of alcoholism in the form of pathological inebriation or dipsomania. The drinker who is prey to the former is dominated by two strong emotions, fear and choleric temper, which occasionally appear in a violent form without any sign of inebriety and may lead to crime. I have been asked for an expert opinion in cases of this kind, and in one of them, which caused a great stir in South Germany a few years ago, my testimony was such that a physician who had murdered his brother-in-law was not prosecuted.

Dipsomania is a kind of intermittent inebriety. It has been described as mental epilepsy, owing to an erroneous interpretation of the symptoms. It is characterized by a state of depressive melancholia of short duration accompanied by a violent craving for alcohol which leads to excesses of the latter. This violent craving for alcohol destined to alleviate the state of depression has its origin in a constitutional anomaly.

A Glance at Alcohol in the Past

Unfortunately we are furnished daily at the present time with a great abundance of documentary evidence regarding the organic and mental alterations due to alcohol. The past supplies no less. Among those men whose names the history of the world has handed down to posterity, among those much more numerous, even countless men who, born in darkness, lived in obscurity and disappeared without leaving more trace than a fleeting shadow, there have been many who, incapable of resisting the passion for drinking spirituous liquors, became victims of the habit, and through their drunkenness brought much evil into the world wherever they had the opportunity or the power.

The history of alcohol is bound up with that of peoples and kings. No human document, however ancient it may be, is old enough to indicate the beginning of the evil. The first users of alcohol were the first to abuse it, because reason and folly are both attributes of human nature and their manifestations are parallel. It is not within everyone's intellectual range to foresee the ends of things and to judge the balance of causes and effects, especially when sensual pleasures and impressions play their part. At all epochs sometimes one people, sometimes another, had the reputation of indulging excessively in the habit of drinking. Documents dating from the primitive ages of humanity, exhortations, legal measures establish the truth of this statement; it is, however, difficult to ascertain whether these measures were directed against the general use of alcohol or merely its abuse.

The Biblical accounts of the effect of alcohol coincide also with our experience. Besides descriptions of grave intoxication and its consequences, at the beginning of the eighth century before our era warnings appear against the injurious consequences of inebriety. They can be found in the Proverbs of Solomon, in Isaiah, Jeremiah, Amos, and Hosea. No doubt drunkenness was far from rare at those times, and its general consequences were well known:

> Wine and women make wise men fall off.
> Woe unto them that rise up early in the morning, that they may follow strong drink; that continue until night, till wine inflame them!

Isaiah refers to drunkards in these words. Without a description of the effects of wine they can even be recognized as such.

Or the biting irony:

> Woe unto them that are mighty to drink wine, and men of strength to mingle strong drink!

The reproach of intemperance was occasionally made against the tribe of Ephraim by the same prophet:

> Woe to the crown of pride, to the drunkards of Ephraim, whose glorious beauty is a fading flower!

Special allusions to its harmful consequences to the organism are also not lacking, for instance with regard to gastric disorders, mobility, disturbances of vision, and hallucinations.

> But they also have erred through wine and through strong drink are out of the way; the priest and the prophet have erred through strong drink, they are swallowed up of wine, they are out of the way through

strong drink; they err envision, they stumble in judgment.

For all tables are full of vomit and filthiness, so that there is no place clean.

Who hath woe? Who hath sorrow? Who hath contentions? Who hath babbling? Who hath wounds without cause? Who hath redness of eyes?

Thine eyes shall behold strange women, and thine heart shall utter perverse things.

The drinker of old made light of the advice of others and the warning signals of his body just as does the drinker of to-day. Punishment and shame do not fright the slave of alcohol:

They strike me, I feel no pain. They beat me, I feel nothing. Then I shall awake and indulge in it (wine) again.

Not only wine but also liquors similar to brandy were employed. The word ⵟⵟ, which is used in Proverbs and in Isaiah, refers to very powerful alcoholic beverages mixed with spices and therefore containing essential oils.

Wherever a substance with the properties of alcohol was discovered, its abuse and the consequences thereof did not fail to appear. In Egypt wine and beer were consumed. The use of both is described in the earliest accounts. The hieroglyph of a wine press already appears, according to Flinders Petrie, in the middle of the First Dynasty under the reign of Den-Semti. Wine was demanded at social meetings. No condemnation of drunkenness occurs before the Nineteenth Dynasty. In the Seventeenth Dynasty a servant asks a guest to drink, to drink to intoxication: "Be of a festive disposition!" And the lady says: "Give me eighteen vessels of wine: you see, I love drunkenness!" The alcoholic beverages of the Egyptians did not lack variety. A glance at the bill of fare on the tombs informs us that the dead demanded no less than six kinds of wine and four of beer. There were many exhortations and warnings to the living and especially to the youth of Egypt, as I have already stated.

With respect to Greece and the Roman Empire, that nauseous fen wherein sat a whole population in churlish and immoral putrefaction, the writers of those times have depicted drunkenness in a hideous but doubtless true manner. In the refined circles of the rich classes drunkenness was more shamefully and repugnantly indulged in than elsewhere at that time.

But Christians too gave rise to scandal by indulging to excess in alcoholic beverages. The apostle St. Paul bears witness that some of them had so little mastery of themselves as to become drunk during the love-feasts celebrated in common. Novatian, the Father of the Church, in the third century speaks of Christians who in the morning, after fasting, began the day by drinking, and poured wine into their still "empty veins," and are drunk before they have eaten. "They do not go to the taverns, but are taverns in themselves, and their pleasure is drinking." And what do the drinking vessels signify which are discovered in the catacombs? They are of glass, and flat, and engraved or painted in gold with pictures of saints, or short inscriptions, such as the names of these saints or "bibe in pace."

Alcohol was and is still abused throughout the world from East to West. In the *Rig-Veda,* which was honoured as a divine revelation, the inebriating drink of the Indian is mentioned, that much-discussed soma,[3] whose mode of preparation has so far not been discovered. I regard soma as a very strong alcoholic beverage obtained by fermentation of a plant worshipped like the plant itself. Sura seems to be a kind of brandy. According to Strabo they drank a wine made from rice instead of barley, which must have been similar to arrack. Distilleries existed at that time which satisfied the taste of the Indians for soma and probably for other alcoholic beverages such as *kilala* and *parisrut.* Drunkenness therefore doubtless existed with all its consequences, the most serious of which were regarded by the sura drinker as "outrages against the gods."

I should only be repeating in different terms what I have already stated if I attempted to describe in detail the state of alcoholism during the succeeding centuries down to the present day. Indeed, nothing has changed with respect to man and his bad instincts, his desires and their outward manifestations. Manners, customs, and dress may change, but the aberrations of moral consciousness, including the faculty of self-judgment, will never disappear from humanity, any more than will the good qualities. The drunkenness of the Germanic tribes, who did not abandon their liking for alcohol after their conversion to Christianity, that of the Goths in the sixth century, that of the Franks at their feasts in which the women also took part, the intemperance not only of the common people but also of the monks and clergy in the ninth century against which Charlemagne issued a capitulary, the alcoholic debauchery of the following centuries, especially the first half of the sixteenth century, the great period of alcoholism in Germany, satirically described by Sebastian Brandt, and finally all that recent centuries have shown us with respect to inebriety firmly establishes the fundamental truth that *abuse is the brother of use*, and it matters little whether this principle be applied to the question of right, power, liberty, love, play, purging and bleeding, eating, or the use of alcoholic beverages. However, in no case does use incline more to abuse than in that of narcotic or stimulating substances. The peculiar influences exercised by alcohol on the functions of the brain on the one hand and individual sensibility on the other explain, as I have already pointed out, the character and range of the injurious effects which result from its abuse, the obstinate perseverance in the vice, and the praise of alcohol even if it brings death. A characteristic example of this last is the epitaph of a drunkard in a church in Florence:

> *Wine, which gives life, to me gave death.*
> *Sober I never saw the dawn—*
> *Now my very bones are thirsty!*
> *Wanderer! Besprinkle the tomb with wine,*
> *Empty the cup, and go!*
> *Farewell, ye drinkers!*

Often social misery gives rise to drunkenness and the latter again to social misery, and to human wretchedness in general where it had not existed before. Whole strata of society may become victims of alcoholism. But the pages of history point out other facts: how the great ones of the earth who were able to exercise a decisive influence on the destiny of mankind have indirectly led individuals or nations to misery or ruin by their drunkenness. This has occurred frequently in such a way that few were unable to perceive the chain of events. But in other cases only the medical specialist is in a position to re-establish the facts and their initial cause. Volumes might be filled with proofs of the influence of alcohol in history from a medical point of view. Antiochus Epiphanes (i.e. the Famous) was called on account of the actions he performed in a state of inebriety, "Epimanes," i.e. the Furious, and was overcome by the Maccabees. Philip of Macedon was a drinker, and his son, Alexander the Great, who was an excessive alcoholic, frequently spent two days and nights in a state of intoxication. He committed many misdeeds during dipsomaniac crises and found through alcohol a premature death. King Antigonus was a drinker, and Dionysius the younger, the Sicilian tyrant, was said to remain in a state of intoxication for three months on end, which resulted in visual disturbances. Darius, the son of Hystaspes, had it inscribed on his tomb that he could drink large amounts of wine without inconvenience:

$$\ldots \; \mathring{\eta} \; \delta \upsilon \nu \acute{\alpha} \mu \eta \nu \; \kappa \alpha \grave{\iota} \; o \mathring{\iota} \nu o \nu \; \pi \acute{\iota} \nu \epsilon \iota \nu \; \pi o \lambda \grave{\upsilon} \nu$$
$$\kappa \alpha \grave{\iota} \; \tau o \mathring{\upsilon} \nu \tau o \nu \; \phi \acute{\epsilon} \rho \epsilon \iota \nu \; \kappa \grave{\alpha} \grave{\iota} \; \mathring{\omega} \varsigma \ldots$$

Tiberius was called Biberius on account of his drinking excesses. Caligula, Claudius, Nero, and probably Trajan also were drinkers. The emperors of the later empire, too, Heliogabalus, Galerius, Maximin, drank to excess, and Jovian succumbed in his chamber to the poisonous effects of carbon monoxide gas during one of his frequent drinking bouts. Other Roman and Byzantine potentates have hardly ever suspected the connection of alcoholism with historical crimes and misdeeds. There have always been crowned drunkards in the world, in France, England, Germany, Russia; King Wenceslaus, son of the Emperor Charles IV, competed with many other monarchs, for instance the Emperor Peter the Great, or Elizabeth of Russia, who drank day and night and was usually drunk. More recently the converted pagan "king" Pomare II, who translated the Bible into Polynesian and constructed a church 712 feet long, went to work with the Bible under one arm and a bottle of rum under the other.

Quite as many drunkards can be encountered among the Popes, for example Alexander V, Sixtus V, Nicholas V, Leo X, and many of those who resided at Avignon. Drunkenness had penetrated at a very early date into the ranks of the clergy, according to the exhortations of Saint Jerome. The councils of Carthage, Tours, Worms, Treves, etc., raised an outcry against this state of affairs. Erasmus of Rotterdam said of his epoch: *Monachorum nihil aliud est, quam facere* (!), *esse, bibere.* And how many of those who, in their day, followed with understanding and sagacity in the Lord's footsteps, how many of those who thanks to their genius created immortal works, must be placed among the drunkards! These true heroes of the world finally paid their tribute to

alcohol with their lives because they acted according to the terms of
the epitaph of Epigonus on a frog who had fallen into a wine-barrel:

> ... Φεύ τινες ὕδωρ
> αἴνουσι, μανίην σώφρονα μαινόμενοι.

Woe unto those who commit the wise folly of drinking water!

Alcoholic Beverages

All these and the many other drinkers of present and past times who
in some way or other exercised an influence on their epoch or the life
of their time which to a greater or lesser degree bears on the present
and the future made and continue to make use of alcoholic beverages
of very different kinds, all of which contained ethyl alcohol. Besides
this other alcohols and numerous substances resulting from the mode
of preparation or intentionally added were also present. Ammianus
Marcellinus reports that the Gauls of the fourth century had no wine
in their country although they eagerly desired it. But they prepared
other beverages which had effects similar to wine: *Vini avidum genus
adfectans ad vini similitudinem multiplices potus*. A large volume would
not suffice to describe the alcoholic beverages of the past and present.
It is nevertheless necessary to give some characteristic examples of
man's contrivances to obtain alcohol. This may convince those who
in their ignorance believe in the possibility of preventing its use.

The variety of the processes applied in the manufacture of alcohol may be based on the three general methods which have been laid
down for the first time in the following pages:

(a) The alcoholic fermentation of sugar. This process is the foundation on which the preparation of mead or honey-beer is based. The
latter is still extensively in use in Abyssinia (Bitōo, Tej of Amhara,
Tadi of Oromo), the Galla countries, and in South-West Africa. In
the first century Pliny mentions mead as a drink consisting of water
and honey. The best wine, he says, is prepared with rain-water which
has been previously set aside for five years. Some people, he says, mix
one-third of rain-water prepared in this way with one-third of fresh or
sometimes boiled water and one-third of old honey. The Edda states
that the dwarfs Fjalar and Galar, after having assassinated the wise
Koasin, mixed his blood with honey and prepared a beverage which
endowed everyone who drank of it with the gift of song. The Scandi-

navians drank mead avidly. They introduced it into England, and because the cup of mead played an important role in the nuptial ceremonies which lasted for thirty days, the first month after marriage was called the "honeymoon." Attila is said to have died on the eve of his wedding from drinking too much mead.

To this class of preparations belongs also a very ancient alcoholic beverage, palm-wine. Herodotus informs us approximately 420 years before our era that peasants brought on ships to Babylon this wine which he calls φοινικήιος οἶνος. Different species of palms indeed secrete a considerable quantity of a sugary juice if incisions are made in the in florescences or the upper part of the stems. A frequent renewal of the incision is necessary, for the irritation due to the wound seems to augment the flow of the juice. This wine is consumed in great quantities in South and Central America, in Africa (in Tunis, on the banks of the Congo, on the west coast, on the upper reaches of the Niger, in Liberia, in the hinterland of Togo, on the coast of the Loango, on the east coast to Somali and Monbuttuland, and in Tanganyika). It is also consumed in Asia, in Ceylon, India, the Philippines, the Carolines, New Guinea, New Caledonia, the Solomon, Gilbert, Marshall, Ladrone Islands, the New Hebrides, Marquesas, etc. The following palms are most frequently employed for the preparation of the beverage: *Raphia vinifera, Elaeis guineensis, Borassus flabelliformis, Arenga saccharifera, Hyphaene coriacea, cocos, Attalea speciosa, Mauritia flexuosa, Phoenix*, the date palm.

The banana is also employed in the countries where it grows, for instance in the African lake district, nera the somerset Nile, in Masailand. The Warundi, for example, daily indulge in excessive drinking of banana-wine.

The agaves are also used for the preparation of alcoholic beverages according to the report of Sahagun, the most important historian of America. These products are called pulque or metl. The saccharine juice is obtained by incisions in the floral stem which is then left to ferment. Several million South Americans, as well as Mexicans, drink pulque.

Instead of agaves the juice of certain cacti is utilized for the preparation of fermented beverages, for instance *cereus giganteus* (drunk by Indians and Mexicans in Sonora and Lower California), *opuntia tuna* (whose produce is called cononche), and *opuntia ficus indica*.

In those regions where the sugar-cane grows it is employed for the same purpose, for instance among the Bangala and the Bashilanga in Africa, where it is called *massanga*, in Surinam, the West Indies, etc. In those countries where nature does not supply succhariferous plants instinct has led man to employ substances whose sugar content was ascertained thousands of years later by science. The peoples which inhabit the country between the Caspian Sea in Mongolia and Eastern Siberia, the Kirghiz, Tekinzes, Buriats, Mongols, Tungus, etc., have long known how to prepare alcoholic beverages whose origin is concealed in the obscurity of the past. They used for this purpose mare's milk, the lactose (sugar of milk) of which is transformed into fermentable sugar. In this way they obtained kumiss with 1.5 to 3 per cent alcohol. The latter is consumed a great deal by the Tekinzes in the oasis of Merv and is called *chal*, in Armenia *mazun*, and in the language of the Tartars *katish*. The Creek Zemarchus who was sent as ambassador by the Emperor Justin II in 568 to the Turkish Khan Dizabulus in Central Asia narrates that during the feast given in his honour large quantities of a barbaric beverage called *kosmos* were consumed. Priscus whom the Emperor Theodosius II sent to Attila also mentions a similar liquor called *kamos*.

In the same manner *kefyr* or other fermentative mycelial symbioses produce alcoholic milk beverages, for instance the Armenian *mazun*.

(b) In all the preparations described hitherto the sugar utilized for the fermentation was already present in the substances employed. The second of the general methods adopted in order to obtain alcoholic beverages consists in the transformation into dextrose or maltose of the starch contained in vegetable matter. This process was unconsciously applied by man from the most ancient times. The oldest plant used with this end in view seems to have been millet, whose cultivation is considered an indication of a state of semi-civilization which was succeeded by the use of the plough. With the aid of *eleusine corocana*, whose starch content is very large, an alcoholic millet beer is prepared, for instance among the A'Sandé of the Congo (*batossi*) sometimes together with sorghum. It is also prepared among the Indians (*bojah* or *bojali*) and in the Mahratta States, in Sikkim (*marva*), from there to the east in Bhutan, between Assam and Tibet in the kingdom of Dharma, and to a lesser degree in Nepal.

A beer prepared from *sorghum vulgare* is extensively employed in Africa. The names given to sorghum are *durrha*, *duchn*, and *mtama*. It is the millet of the Negroes, the Moore, and the Kaffirs. The beverage is already consumed on the banks of the upper Nile (*bilbil merissa*), in East Africa, in Somaliland as inebriating liquor, *pombe*, and in a non-inebriating form as *togwa*, in Harar (*bôsa, kuhîja*), Abyssinia (*dalla, soa*), in the Congo territory (*pombe, bussera, malafu*), and southward to the Portuguese possessions, in the Sudan (*merissa, dawa, bosa*), and in South Africa (*oala, boyaloa*).

Probably more recent than millet-beer is that prepared from barley, which seems to have originated in Egypt and in the course of thousands of years spread more and more to the west and north. Strabo states that the Ethiopians still employed it with millet. At the beginning of the seventh century Isidore of Seville writes in his *Origines* of the use of barley as a substitute for wine in Spain. The oldest beer was prepared without hops. In the German monasteries the fabrication of beer was also improved with respect to the keeping properties of the beverage. Barley was chiefly employed, as its name indicates, for according to Grimm *bere* is the ancient Saxon name for barley. In old High German it is *pior*, in Norse *eolo*, in Anglo-Saxon "ale" and "beer." The use of beer as a daily beverage was quite general in the monasteries. Towns had their breweries and malthouses, for instance the town of Freiburg had in 1653 six of the latter and twelve of the former. Especially in the sixteenth century the civil and ecclesiastical courts rivalled the private breweries in the manufacture of beer. In the towns there were primitive house-breweries for the use of the inhabitants and of strangers. In some towns, for instance Hamburg and Lübeck, beer was prepared from wheat and called "white beer." The following figures will convey an idea of the magnitude of the consumption of beer in various countries at the present day. In London about a million and a half quarts of English beer are consumed daily. In Bavaria the consumption is estimated at two hundred and twenty litres per head annually. In all Germany five thousand million litres are manufactured every year.

In distant countries, for example Tibet, a mild beer called *chang* is prepared from barley. This is distilled and a very strong product, arrack, is obtained, not to be confounded with the rum of the same name.

Among the Dyaks of Borneo (*tuak*), in Formosa, and to a very large extent in Japan, rice is employed for the manufacture of alcohol by fermentation. It is stated that *sake* or rice-wine was prepared so long as 2,600 years ago. Detailed reports of its use are forthcoming from the year 90 B.C. The transformation of the starch of rice into sugar and its alcoholic fermentation are due to certain yeast-cells and hyphomycetes (*koji*). In China *sake* is also employed. In Pekin there are rice-wine breweries.

Central and South America have their own particular alcoholic beverages. In these countries it is maize which is utilized for the purpose of obtaining alcohol. It is first boiled, then masticated or chewed. The masticated substance is placed in large earthenware pots, covered with leaves, and left to ferment. Reports of this process date from the year 1526. The use of this maize-beer, *chicha* and *cangüi*, extends from Mexico to Guatemala, Yucatan, and Darien to the high plateau of Bogotà in the south, and is also found among the inhabitants of the Andes, in Ecuador, Peru and Chile to Araucania and eastwards from the Orinoco, and in Guiana as far as the territory of the Amazon. It is the national beverage of the Indians of the Guarani group, especially the Abas or Chiriguanos, and the half-civilized Indians of the Andes, the Quichuas, Aymara, Coroados, etc. Here the manufacturing process consists in the transformation of the maize-starch into dextrine and sugar and the fermentation of the latter. A yellowish, sourish, and fairly inebriating liquid is thus obtained resembling new wine. During the period of Christianization of Peru, etc., exhortations as to the abuse of chicha formed a large part of the sermons of the missionaries. "Chichinism" is not a special disease, but a grave form of alcoholism due to the substances contained in the beverage. Certain peculiar morbid states following on the drinking of chicha, as for instance the frequently observed spots on the hands, occasionally also occur after the consumption of other alcoholic beverages.

The Indians who speak the Quichua language in the mountainous territory of Ecuador prepare their beer from maize (*asua*) by boiling and crushing the plant, which, placed in hermetically sealed receptacles, furnishes sugar and afterwards alcohol through the action of ferments present in the substance.

Another method of obtaining alcoholic beverages has been adopted in South America. *Jatropha manihot*, the kassava tree, contains a large amount of starch, which is known as mandioca, tapioca, or Brazilian arrowroot, as well as a juice rich in hydrocyanic acid. This juice is pressed out and removed and the starch is transformed into sugar ready for fermentation. Here we have another instance where we must admire the ingenuity of the primitive instinct of man which taught him this method of manufacture long before it was scientifically explained. The natives boil the mandioca, the women chew the substance and spit it into a receptacle. The saliva transforms the starch into sugar and the ferments transform the sugar into alcohol. The resulting beverage is called *paiwari* or *paiva* in British Guiana, *taroba* on the Tapajós, *caysúma* in Ega, *cachiri* among the Roucouyennes, *cauim* or *pajuarú* among the aborigines of Brazil. The use of this beverage extends eastward from the territory to the west of the Magdalena to about 50 degrees west longitude, northward to the Caribbean Sea and south to the Amazon and the upper reaches of the Tapajós.

The transformation of starch into sugar by means of saliva is also practised among other isolated tribes, for instance in Formosa with rice and in South America with *yucca*, probably *Yucca angustifolia* (*Yucca glauca, Yucca filamentosa*).

This plant is frequently used for food as well as for the preparation of a very popular beverage. For many tribes, the Jibáros and the Canelos Indians in the east of Ecuador, for instance, the Cholones on the upper reaches of the Huallaga, etc., yucca-beer plays a more important part than does the algorobo-beer for the chaco Indians or maize-beer for the Chiriguanos and the Quichuas. The fruit is boiled; it would seem that the Cholones employ the root. A part of the boiled substance is chewed by the women on specially appointed days and thoroughly triturated with saliva; the remainder is merely crushed. The whole mass is then placed in an earthenware jug and left to ferment. In twenty-four hours it is ready for use. It is drunk diluted with water. The Indian on his wanderings carries some of the yucca-substance with him wrapped in banana leaves. By adding water he obtains a mildly inebriating beer of a colour similar to milk which enables him to go without food in cases of emergency. This beverage is consumed at certain drinking feasts. On these occasions the Indian reveals not only his taste for this beverage but also his peculiar religious conceptions.

These conceptions are attached to certain ceremonies as well as to
the beverage itself. During the fermentation of the substance in the
earthenware jugs Karsten observed Indian women squatting round the
vessels singing magic chants which are said to contribute to the success of the process. Later, while the chicha, yucca-beer, or other similar beverages are imbibed, dancing and singing ceremonies of various
kinds take place. They begin before the onset of inebriety sets in and
are continued during the drunken state.

The Indians of Ecuador in the same way prepare a beer from the
fruit of the chonta-palm *Guilelma speciosa* (the *chuntáruru* of the
Canelos Indians, the *ui* of the Jibáros) which they cultivate. The preparation and consumption of this beer are likewise accompanied by ceremonies.

Another substance which furnishes an alcoholic beverage is the
algorobo from the fruits of the leguminous plants *Prosopis alba, Prosopis
pallida,*[4] *Prosopis juliflora*. The Indians of Ecuador, Paraguay, and the
northern parts of the Argentine—all the tribes of the Gran Chaco—
impatiently await the ripening of the fruits, which also serve as an
important food. The Matacos, Chorotis, Ashluslay, etc., have all kinds
of ceremonies for the chasing away of evil spirits who may impede the
ripening of the plant. The ripe seeds with the pulp of the fruit are
masticated and mixed with saliva. After being soaked in very hot water the substance is left to ferment in a goatskin. This process is accompanied by chanting and the beating of drums in order to drive
away harmful demons. The men alone drink the product to complete
inebriety. The same results are obtained from a beer of *Acacia aroma*
(*tusca*) or *Gourliea decorticans* (*chañar*), a fruit tree with plum-like fruits,
or *Tizyphus mistol* (*mistol*), whose fruits, resembling over-ripe grapes,
are prepared in the way already indicated, by being masticated and
mixed with saliva. All these beverages are considered to increase physical strength in a marked manner.

We must now leave these primitive alcoholic beverages of distant
countries, whose only European analogy would seem to be the Russian kvas, prepared by acid and alcoholic fermentation from wheat,
rye, barley, buckwheat flour, and bread, and pass on to other beverages used in various lands, consisting of purer and more concentrated
alcohol.

(c) The third method, the distillation of alcoholic liquors, answers to a more advanced scientific development. In those cases where this method was employed by Asiatic peoples of an inferior degree of civilization they probably gained the knowledge from Europeans or in some cases even from the Chinese. Weak alcoholic beverages did not give satisfaction, and were replaced by spirits.

The Buryats drug themselves with milk-spirits obtained by distillation. The Kalmuks and Tartars make use of an arrack prepared from milk. The Tekinzes of the oasis of Merv employ *chal*, a product of the distillation of camel's or cow's milk, which is suitably treated.

In the Far East large quantities of rice-spirit are manufactured. The name of this beverage in China is *samshu*.[5] According to whether it has been distilled once, twice, or three times it is called *Mei Chau (Leu Pun Chau)*, *Sheung Ching Chau*, or *Sam Ching Chau*. Its alcoholic content varies from 50 to 60 per cent. The Chinwan of Formosa, the Gilyaks, the Kakhyen of the Khasia mountains, and many other tribes make use of this intoxicant. A Chinese spirit is also prepared from millet, usually *Sorghum vulgare*. Special factories in Manchuria produce more than two million vedro of *chanshin* every year. In some districts the people prepare it at home with primitive implements. On account of their cheapness these spirits, defying all interdictions, have penetrated into the Amur and Transbaikal territory. It is said that this beverage produces two inebriations. On the day following the consumption of a large quantity of the spirit intense thirst is experienced, and on drinking a glass of water a second state of inebriation supervenes, more violent and of longer duration than the first. Chinese spirits contain a considerable amount of fusel oil. We find in different parts of the earth an innumerable variety of distilled spirits for its many hundred million people. Where potatoes, corn, grapes, etc., are not available man takes other substances containing starch or sugar and prepares distilled spirits by extremely primitive means. In Central Asia, for instance, besides rice, *Sorghum vulgare* is utilized, its seeds serving the Karens of Burma for the preparation of spirits. Less known plants, however, are also employed for this purpose. The inhabitants of Kamchatka manufacture a very powerful distilled product resembling spirits from *Heracleum spondylium*, hogweed, by letting the stems ferment. The natives of Honolulu use the roots of *Cordyline terminalis* (*tishualh*) to the same end. The Tahitians, the natives of the Tuba and Sandwich Islands, and the Maoris employ *Cordyline australis*, or more often at the present day bread-fruit, pineapple, and orange juice. The inhabitants of Tasmania use the berries of *Cissus antarctica*, the Hottentots the fruits of the *Grewia* species, the Indians the blossoms of *Bassia latifolia* (*mahwá, mahua*). The Indians of Eastern Ecuador obtain an alcoholic liquor from the distillation of roasted yucca fruits. In Germany and other countries *Sorbus aucuparia*, rowan, *Sambucus*, etc., are occasionally used.

The other artificial preparations on a basis of more or less pure alcohol manufactured in civilized countries and also in use in noncivilized areas are extremely varied mixtures containing essential oils or other substances. Their stimulating effects on the palate and the brain differ in character and intensity. For the most part they contain many injurious secondary substances (fusel oil, aldehydes, furfurol, etc.) so that they play an extremely important part from the toxicological standpoint when their use is chronic and the individual limits of resistance have been exceeded. This may be said of absinthe, a beverage now prohibited in France, an alcoholic solution of essential oil of absinthe. The countless drinks mixed by bartenders are frequently nothing other than alcoholic solutions of essential oils. These beverages are also prepared at the counter by women, who, like the Circe of Homer, transform men into pigs. Eau de Cologne is used by drinkers in Africa (Tabora, Zanzibar), British India, America, and Europe. It is even preferred to rum, brandy, and other liquors of the same kind. A liquor prepared with *Capsicum annuum*, Cayenne pepper, should be included here. It appears to have a very distressing influence on the drinker.

To some Chinese beverages the root of *Sophoratomentosa*, which contains cytisine, is added. This has very exciting properties. It is stated that in the district of San Antonio (Texas) the Indians used and still use the seeds of *Sophora secundiflora* in doses of half a seed in order to become intoxicated. A state of gaiety is succeeded, according to reports, by two to three days of sleep.

With the aid of *Epilobium angustifolium* and many other plants alcoholic beverages are prepared all the world over, which exercise diverse influences on the brain. They all contain, besides alcohol, other substances, essential oils, etc., which reinforce or modify the injurious action of the alcohol.

I have described the action of alcohol on the development of fertilized eggs. Table 7 shows how essential oils of the kind mentioned above influence this development.

TABLE 7. INFLUENCE OF THE INJECTION OF ALCOHOLIC SOLUTIONS OF ESSENTIAL OILS ON THE DEVELOPMENT OF EGGS

NUMBER OF EGGS	SUBSTANCE INJECTED	NORMAL	NOT DEVELOPED	ABNORMAL
24	Ethyl Alcohol	62.50	16.66	20.83
24	Alcoholic Solution of Anise Oil	41.66	25.00	33.33
24	Alcoholic Solution of Absinthe Oil	16.66	21.43	62.50

Certain conclusions may be drawn from this table. In practice its immediate significance for man is not very large. However, it may always be asserted that the effect of alcohol on a drinker is more noxious if essential oils are added which are liable to act in a different manner from the alcohol itself. If such extremely injurious substances as nitrobenzene are added to spirits in order to render them more intoxicating and palatable, we must regard it as a deplorable practice from every point of view. It is claimed that on account of its furfurol and higher alcoholic content brandy is more injurious in animal experiments than ethyl alcohol.

The aggravating effects due to the presence of essential oils in addition to alcohol have been experimentally ascertained hundreds of years ago. It was discovered that if rosmarine was added to beer during its manufacture a product was obtained which gave rise not only to headache but even to stupor. From early Roman times to the seventeenth century so-called mixed wines (i.e. wines which had added to them essential oils from organic material such as rosmarine, fennel, anise, absinthe, euphrasy, sage, and hyssop) were consumed. Claret is such an aromatic wine. It is prepared from honey, clove, grains of paradise (*Amomum melegueta rosc.*), cinnamon bark, and ginger. In the eighteenth century the famous drink hippocrass was still made from wine with cinnamon, pimento, clove, nutmeg, ginger, and pieces of greengages; or sometimes with the addition of almonds, musk, and amber. Pliny states that in the beginning of the Roman Empire not only were aromatic plants employed in the manufacture of perfumed wines, but also the evil Mandragora, which suffices by itself to produce a state of somnolence. The action on the brain of these aromatic wines (*vina odoure condita*) which are still used at the present day is an unpleasantly reinforced alcoholic action, even if the effects are not experienced immediately.

It is therefore not only the quantity which in the long run injures the body and the soul of the drunkard, but also, and to an even greater extent, the composition of the beverage. Some kinds of wine are even more noxious than certain spirits. One wine of this kind, the *Est* of Montefiascone, will never be forgotten. The nobleman Johann von Fugger, who was a drunkard, caused a servant always to ride in advance of him and write on the door of every tavern where he found good wine *Est* (here!). At Montefiascone he wrote *Est* three times. His master arrived, and drank so much that he died. On his tomb, which is said to be still in existence, the following words were inscribed by his servant:

> *Est, est, est, propter nimium est*
> *Dominus meus mortuus est.*
>
> *Here, here, here, too much of this "here"*
> *My master drank, so now he lies here.*

Temperance and Abstinence

In the preceding pages I have given a sufficiently clear and precise description of my conception of alcoholism. It is founded on toxicology, on what I have myself seen and my own experiences as an expert. It is unnecessary to copy statistical records of the increase of alcoholism in civilized and savage countries and its harmful effects on the people, or to lay stress on its well-known social consequences, domestic misery, poverty, degradation, and so on. The far-reaching import of this evil is clear to everyone, without further explanation; it is clear also that if alcoholism were abolished some little happiness would be created despite the continuance of many even greater miseries on earth.

No period of history has been free from attempts to combat alcoholism on a larger or smaller scale. Individuals and groups addressed its devotees in the language of religion, common sense and reason, and by means of laws and regulations. They even attempted altogether to suppress alcohol for consumption. For the reasons which I set forth when dealing with morphia these efforts were of little or no avail, with the exception of those of Mohammedanism, which for several centuries kept its believers from alcohol but could not prevent the use of equivalent substances. Moreover, the words of Mohammed are nowadays frequently vain on account of the spread of civilization and the influence of Western modes of living on the Orient. The mighty energy of the powerful modern alcoholic beverages has vanquished the instructions of the Prophet. It is therefore not improper to speak of an increasing alcoholization of the Orient, even if we admit that popular belief still considers the use of alcohol as an infringement of the law. The same is the case with the Hindus. This people is naturally sober and temperate. No decent Hindu will drink spirits, which are as rigorously prohibited as is, for instance, the eating of beef. Nevertheless, here also alcohol and many other substances which should not have made their way have overturned ancient custom. The Methodist sect also practices complete abstinence from alcoholic beverages.

At the present day the ancient and multiform combat against alcoholism shows itself in a new form. It is directed chiefly against alcohol in itself. By "psycho-scientific" processes all its physiological effects are transformed into sins. Minute experiments prove that not only is drunkenness an evil, but that everyone who drinks alcohol in whatever quantity is a dangerous person. The band of abstainers, though as old as the world itself, was formerly not a very large one. At the present day it has become more important, and many of its members, convinced apostles of its principles, carry forth in speech and in writing the gospel of abstinence.

I respect those who for one reason or another abstain from alcohol just as I do those who live in conformity with religious prescriptions, such as the observance of Ramadan, the Mohammedan month of fasting, the keeping of a vow or some form of asceticism, vegetarianism, antinicotinism, etc. It is a private matter for the individual, as is the abstinence from alcohol. The individual may have his own reasons for its justification, just as he may have for not eating such and such a food. But to condemn the general effects of alcohol and to convert others to this opinion more is needed than subjective reasons, even more than we can read in books and pamphlets. To the majority of abstainers who feel themselves bound to an apostolate, the following words of Lessing can be applied: "Who is there, who, when he believes himself to be enlightened, does not desire to enlighten others? The most ignorant, the greatest fools, exhibit the greatest ardour. This may be seen at all times. A shallow brain gets some vague notion of a science or an art, and babbles of it on all occasions."

In this sphere, as in others in our days, suggestive slogans are employed. "Pay by Post" is inscribed in lapidary letters on the post office. Patent bed manufacturers tell us to "Sleep Patent," gas companies to "Cook with Gas!", shoe factories adjure us "No more Cold Feet!" Why "No more Alcohol!"? It is nothing but a slogan, a mere phrase. Why such an expenditure of efforts against alcohol alone, where there are other deeper cravings which well deserve some apostolic effort? Why is there no general crusade against morphia, cocaine, nicotine, caffeine, lust, gambling? The anti-alcoholic fight is based on no clear judgment; it is conducted with party-spirit. Its leaders are for the most part laymen, though professors of medicine also take part in it. But when these latter have once adopted an erroneous point of view their obstinacy is unrivalled. No opinion can be derived from psychological investigations, but only from science, a science founded on the observation of facts; and this, as I have already stated, is lacking.

We smile at the reasons given in ancient times for total abstinence from alcohol. Certain Christian sects, the Encratites, the Tatianists, the Marcionites, and the Water-drinkers, considered the consumption of wine a sin; the Servians said that the devil after having been expelled from heaven transformed himself into a snake and mixed with the earth, the product of this mixture being the vine. The stems, the snake-like arms of the vine proved its diabolic origin. But it is more than ridiculous to state at the present day that alcohol is "poison for the human race which eventually leads to the degeneration of whole classes of society," or that it is "in all circumstances a poison in the ordinary sense of the word," or even that "the consumption of a single glass of wine or beer diminishes the intellectual faculties," that "alcohol shortens life in general and especially that part of it which is economically profitable." The greatest nonsense of all, manifesting the supremest ignorance of the facts, is the statement that "the life of abstemious persons is of longer duration than that of even moderate drinkers," and so on.

Were this so, the compelling question arises: to whom does the world of to-day owe its form and its activity, to abstainers or to nonabstainers? To the latter alone, without doubt. They have been the creators and promoters of science. To them we owe the beautiful creations of art. They have supplied the wonderful feats of the poetic imagination, and the noble productions of music have been forthcoming from the profound depths of their sensibility. They have discovered by calculation the presence of new worlds in the far-off spaces of the universe, and later on even perceived them. Their ingenuity solved for them many enigmas posed by the existence of things, and they have foretold the present and the future as if informed by a divine inspiration. Non-abstainers launched speech on its journey across terrestrial space on the waves of the ether. Zealous and inspired with the joy of discovery they have opened roads on this globe which but for them would never have been trodden. Even if among this multitude of the elect one or another, through bodily weakness, has renounced alcohol, what is this in comparison with all the others who are indebted to this stimulant not only for hours of joy but frequently for the impulse to their contribution to the well-being of mankind?

It is incomprehensible and indefensible that abstainers should consider a man who has a liking for wine as an inferior creature. Even if he drinks it in considerable quantities there is not the least reason for this view, especially when he has given precious and lasting gifts to mankind. The Apostle Paul says: "Let not him that eateth despise him that eateth not; and let not him which eateth not judge him that eateth." A Heidelberg mathematician once told me the following story. One day as he was ascending the Schlossberg with a Heidelberg philosopher the latter suddenly left his side because he did not want to pass before the statue of a drunkard. The "drunkard" was no other than Victor von Scheffel! We also read that Goethe was possessed with the demon of alcohol. This is said to be the reason why his family after the third generation was destined to become extinct. This is the false invention of an ignorant and fanatical abstainer. Even were it true, however, the name "Goethe" of itself would transform into praise the accusation of incurable imbecility hurled at wine-drinkers, just as in the Scriptures water was transformed into wine by Jesus, who was also Himself accused of drunkenness because he appreciated wine. As a matter of fact, Goethe's son inherited alcoholism from his grandfather, Vulpius, whose drunkenness reduced his family to misery, and who frequently pawned his clothes to obtain money for drinking. Goethe's wife, Christiane Vulpius, in later years gave many proofs of her pernicious inheritance. His son August followed her example to such an extent that he deserved the name of drunkard. Frau von Stein reports that one evening he drank seventeen glasses of champagne at a club.

In my capacity as pharmacologist and toxicologist I wholly reject those experiments which have led certain psycho-physicians to conclude that alcohol in any quantity, however small, intoxicates the brain. Such experiments may be very interesting, but their value is completely insignificant when compared to the facts of common knowledge which are the result of everyday experience of the effects of alcohol in moderate doses. These psychophysical experiments can be compared, for instance, to the experimental treatment of healthy subjects with homœopathic medicines. In both cases the tests are carried out on persons who, merely because they were subjects of the experiments, were under the influence of suggestion and therefore wished to furnish interesting reports. The numerous symptoms, among them grave organic disorders, which are said to have appeared after homœopathic treatment with water that had for some time been in contact with pure gold should be considered in the light of the fact that millions of persons permanently carry gold in their mouths in the form of fillings or crowns for their teeth. But I would go further, and declare that if errors due to suggestion were ignored, the experiments made to ascertain the action of small quantities of alcohol on the brain with respect to the fundamental character of the personality, the capacity for work, excitability, resistance to fatigue, etc., are valid only for their subjects.

Those psychologists who come to other conclusions are in my opinion ignorant of real life. They should, as I have been doing for more than twenty years, observe and investigate the different degrees and varieties of individual sensibility to alcohol, of skilled and ordinary workmen in factories. If the output of work before and after the consumption of three-tenths of a litre of beer were measured, nothing or very little of the results of the so-called general psychological experiments made on a few individuals would remain valid. And this is just the quantity of beer, according to the psychological decision, which, after an initial diminution of the mental reaction, gives rise to dullness of the perceptive faculties. Thousands of brain-workers drink wine of an evening without experiencing, apart from an appreciable brain-stimulation, any "paralysing" effects. The statement that the effects of alcohol, which are usually considered as the effects of excitation (mental excitation, amplification of the output of the heart, suppression of the feeling of fatigue, etc.) are all fundamentally phenomena of paralysis, violates the most elementary truths of biology. It is absurd to attribute a paralysing effect to alcohol and even more so to attempt to support this assumption by elaborate experiments. It is a source of error both for medical men unskilled in pharmacology and for the general public. They have the impression that these experiments are constants, whereas they are, as I have explained, nothing but unimportant investigations on biased and easily influenced subjects.

To believe that the effects of ethyl alcohol on the psyche are the same in all individuals is a fundamental error. This assertion is without any foundation in the case of those who take, even daily, a moderate dose of alcohol, provided it is kept within the limits which their individual sensibility permits them to tolerate, and it is only of relative significance in the case of those who exceed these limits. Perusal of my work on the secondary effects of medicinal substances will show that on every page there are facts to prove that the influence of personality renders illusory every fixation or preconceived determination of the effects on the body of a chemical substance.

It is a general opinion of abstainers, which has become an axiom, that alcohol paralyses the higher mental functions, diminishes the quality of intellectual work, the sharpness and accuracy of conception, the clearness of judgment, and the faculties of memory. We must refute this opinion not only on account of the importance of the personal factor, but also on the grounds stated above. While no one will doubt that it holds good for a person in a state of drunkenness, in this general and apodictic form it is not even applicable to a drinker or a drunkard. I have already pointed out the irrelevance of psychological experimental methods which claim to prove the deteriorating effect of small doses of alcohol on the brain, for instance in the following manner. Is a person capable of learning by heart 25 verses of the Odyssey after taken 25 c.c. of alcohol? I am sure that even without alcohol I should be incapable of accomplishing this feat, although I have an excellent memory for facts in my own special sphere of knowledge and in kindred sciences, such as chemistry, physics, botany, and history. As for experiments carried out on abstemious persons who consumed half a liter of wine, corresponding to two liters of beer, where a retardation in the process of adding up figures, a greater difficulty in learning by heart, etc., appeared for a period of 12 to 24 or even 48 hours, I consider these as only significant of the personal state of the subjects and nothing more. These cases are just as interesting as a paradoxical fever produced by the action of quinine, diarrhœa after opium, parotitis in certain lead-workers, cutaneous eruptions after consumption of mushrooms, or syncope after smelling a flower which for other persons has an agreeable odour. In the great majority of cases the cerebral effects of alcohol taken in small doses are so transient and momentary that it is a matter of daily experience that there can be practically no question of any important disadvantage resulting therefrom.

The conclusion to which I arrive is as follows. Prohibition, for instance, as it is compulsorily enforced by law in the United States of America, cannot be defended by recourse to accurate scientific psychological research nor by the testimony of physical disturbances produced by the moderate use of alcohol. In spite of all this abstainers act just as subjectively as certain Christian sects did nearly two thousand years ago, who celebrated Holy Communion with water. They are influenced by individual aversion to or fear of alcohol and its consequences—the same reasons that bring about abstinence from tobacco. There is really objective reason for their abstinence.

Between excess and abstention lies temperance. The efforts made by temperance societies to prevent the abuse of strong spirits have given rise to a flood of propaganda, among it much that is extremely weak in argument. It has been forthcoming from "social hygienists" who know very little of hygiene and still less of the course of the effects of alcohol, and who are far from knowing the conditions of life of the working classes, so that they are not in a position to favour the world with their lucubrations. It is useless to dwell on the well-established reasons for temperance. Temperance is a vital necessity. It should consequently be applied as a law of life to the satisfaction of all man's desires. Temperance excludes the craving, or at least prevents it from reaching morbidity. Therefore writings in favour of alcoholic temperance must excite our sympathy even though we consider that their utility is not in proportion to the trouble and labour expended on them.

Nevertheless, these writings contrast favorably with the conditions created in recent years in America by the prohibition laws, especially by the Volstead Act and the Eighteenth Amendment to the Constitution, against which, in 1919, President Wilson opposed his veto in vain. At the present day, the manufacture, sale, and transportation of alcoholic beverages, as well as their import and export, are prohibited in the United States of America. Permits are, however, granted to medical men, who are allowed to prescribe whiskey or wine for their patients if they think it necessary. Not more than a pint may be allowed to the same patient within a period of ten days. It is alleged that 45,000 physicians made use of this permission and issued 13,800,000 alcohol permits in a single year. According to reports of the apparently well-established alcohol traffic in the United States in 1925, many former innkeepers and waiters in the character of qualified pharmacists have opened up new pharmacies for the sale of whiskey. The number of pharmacies in New York State increased from 1,565 in the year 1916 to 5,190 in the year 1922, and has since then further increased in proportion. These whiskey-pharmacies sell legitimate wares below their usual price in order to attract customers for their whiskey trade. During my travels in America from ocean to ocean I made many observations and investigations in the "dry States." I came to the conclusion that there exists an enormous amount of anti-alcoholic propaganda of a most unpleasant kind. Compulsory abstinence has reached such a point that those who have not recently observed the state of affairs with their own eyes would hardly believe it possible that the law could be publicly flouted so frequently and openly and with such gay insolence that the ironic question of foreigners, "When are you going to introduce prohibition?" seems perfectly justified.

If, on the other hand, we read the official American reports on the results of prohibition we might believe that a veritable golden age is reigning in that country. According to these reports, general prosperity has increased, savings-bank deposits have been augmented, the output of manual labour is larger and better, accidents are less frequent, business has increased, and purchasing power is greater. More books are bought, more magazines are read, and more milk is drunk. Prostitution has decreased, adultery is less frequent, venereal diseases and suicides are diminishing, infantile mortality is declining, murder, assaults, robberies, thefts and even pocket-picking have diminished by 30 to 80 per cent, as well as arrests for vagrancy and drunkenness. This last, however, showed an increase in 1921 and 1922. The alcohol-psychosis decreased by 50 per cent in certain parts, and the number of deaths due to alcohol diminished in the years 1916 to 1920 by 84 per cent in fourteen large cities, etc. All that is now necessary in this country is for the blessings of prohibition to bring about the realization of the words of Isaias: "The wolf also shall dwell with the lamb, and the leopard shall lie down with the kid; the calf and the young lion and the fatling together; and a little child shall lead them." If, as a contrast, the statistics of criminality for New York City are examined, assuming that they are accurate, they produce a very different impression by reason of their disproportion with the facts cited on the preceding pages. The number of murders whose perpetrators were for the greater part undiscovered, amounted to 237 in 1921, 262 in 1923, and 333 in 1924. In 1924 there were 7,000 cases of housebreaking before the courts of which only 587 ended with a conviction.

As the use of alcoholic beverages has, for the greater part of mankind, become a vital necessity, the desire to procure alcohol inevitably leads to infringements of the law, fraud, smuggling, etc., especially in the "dry States." This year many persons were incriminated in an affair of this kind in Cleveland.

Grave exaggerations of the effects of alcohol, although their bias is manifest, do not fail to find many fanatic and obstinate believers. To these exaggerations we may oppose the following statement, the fruit of the experience of many years. There is no state of moral inferiority in a people which can be attributed to any one single cause, as in this instance alcohol. It is not possible to imagine any means, even the complete annihilation of all the alcohol in the world, which would bring about in so short a space of time such prodigious progress on the way of perfection as is claimed by the reports quoted. These exaggerations are probably the invention of fervent admirers of the new American alcohol legislation. This legislation strikes with the same interdict the just man and the sinner, the man who is always conscious of the limits of his individual capacity for alcohol and the inveterate drunkard. However, this prohibition exists only on paper. And this country has been emancipated from alcohol, and is an example to the whole world for all time! No! Not forever, for I fancy that this fanatical prohibition has roused adverse forces which will one day be able to restore things to a reasonable level.

No! The idea that the world can be improved by innovations of this kind is destitute of all reasonable foundation. The quantities of alcohol which a person with normally inhibitory senses consumes are neither physically nor intellectually injurious. He is beneficially affected by them quite apart from the alimentary qualities of alcohol. Saint Clement of Alexandria knew the Biblical estimation of the virtues of wine, and knew also that no Sabbath and no festival of the Jews passes without the utterance of the words of benediction and thanksgiving for the fruit of the vine before meals:

> Blessed art Thou, O Lord our God, King of the Universe, Who hast created the fruit of the vine!

Saint Clement glorifies wine because it improves the temper, clears the judgment, brings harmony into our intercourse with strangers and servants, and makes us more benevolent towards friends. However, wine has other properties. Ever since man has been in possession of it, it has proved a friend to countless numbers of wretched beings in their times of spiritual misery. In the hour of sorrow and grief it has brought joy to their hearts. In solitude, anxiety, and fear, it has restored their equilibrium. It has effaced frowns from their brows, dispensed calm to the hopeless, the embittered and the desperate, and enabled all to catch a glimpse for an hour or two of the rosy-fingered dawn of a new and better day. Into the heart of those sufferers for whom no joyous hour seems ever to strike, it appears for a short space the balm of releasing forgetfulness. In the dying, it has frequently stayed the departing soul long enough to permit his lips to utter some important word or farewell.

The great oracle once declared that Socrates was the wisest of men, and this sage expressed himself as follows:

> It seems to me, O friends, to be right to drink; for wine comforts the soul, soothes the sorrow of man like mandragora, and arouses joy as oil the flame.
>
> ... ἀλλὰ πίνειν μὲν, ὦ ἄνδρες, καὶ ἐμοὶ πάνυ δοκεῖ, τῷ γὰρ ὄντι ὁ οἶνος ἄρδων τὰς ψυχὰς, τὰς μὲν λύπας, ὥσπερ ὁ μανδράγορας, ἀνθρώπους, κοιμίζει. τὰς δὲ φιλοφροσύνας ὥσπερ ἔλαιον φλόγας ἐγείραι.

What was the opinion of the later ages? In all times clear-sighted people have recognized that a reasonable and moderate consumption of wine is not harmful, but that drunkenness is an evil. A great sage of the twelfth century, Maimonides, pointed out that not everyone is able to make proper use of wine; that if taken immoderately it is an evil, because inebriety is a disorder of the brain, and that young people should abstain from it, but that young people should abstain from it, but that it is of value for the old. It is a kind of prophylactic for the conservation of old age. It is necessary to make some reservations with respect to the latter statement, as well as to the description of Ambroise Paré[6] several centuries later: "L'eau de vie, une espcèe de panacée, dont les vertus sont infinies," but their opinions contain some truth. The medical man considers alcohol a valuable remedy in case of need, and many laymen are of the same opinion. When Achille Ratti, the present Pope Pius XI, an experienced Alpinist, had ascended the Dufourspitze, he suffered from cold and fatigue. The wine and eggs having frozen, he and his companion resorted to chocolate and the remains of some "excellent kirschwasser."[7] From a pharmacological point of view they were perfectly right.

In striking contrast to all these benefits are the repugnant pictures of drunkenness, which Montaigne[8] describes as "vice lasche et stupide," with its troubles of physical and mental co-ordination. But if all these benefits are correct (and it is only from a sectarian and partisan point of view that they can be doubted) then let us, while pitying the drunkard, make allowances for the temperate man who for once has gone astray from the path of decency. It is not to be borne that those who know how to remain within the limits of moderation should be treated as "inferior creatures" only because they drink wine.

An abstainer is not a superior being simply because he renounces alcohol, just as the person who has taken a vow of chastity may not consider himself better than another who obeys the normal impulses of his nature. The same is the case with abstainers from tobacco who are not subject to the occasionally harmful by-effects of nicotine, but do not experience the agreeable feeling of relaxation which accompanies the smoking of a pipe or a cigar. Abstinence may be justified as an individual conviction, but not a gospel.

Conclusion

In the prodigiously complex activity of the universe whereof human life is but a minute part, man's power is infinitely small. And if he has the gift of exercising an influence, it can be but within very modest limits, and only on the innate or acquired instincts of the individual. Man under certain conditions can tame lions, tigers or bears, bring certain herbivores to consume meat, or make some inferior organisms change over for some time from salt to fresh water, but he can only succeed if the means at his disposal have a far greater energy than the instincts to be overcome. It is possible for a certain time to prevent the criminal from exercising his antinomian impulses by imprisonment. It is possible officially to declare an alcoholic incapable of managing his affairs. But, according to experience as old as the world itself, none of these measures has any lasting effect. The permanent cure of an alcoholic is, with very few exceptions, improbable.

None of the many regulations and punishments which from the oldest times to the present day have been enforced against drunkenness and alcoholism have had the slightest positive result. A few examples suffice to prove this. In ancient Rome, as well as at Miletus and Massilia (Marseilles) women were not allowed to drink wine. The wife of Egnatius Mecenius, who had drunk wine from a barrel, was beaten to death by her husband, who was acquitted by Romulus. Pompilius Faunus had his wife scourged to death because she had emptied a pot of wine. Another Roman woman of title was condemned to die of hunger merely because she had opened the cupboard containing the keys of the wine-cellar. The men of western Locri, the first prohibitionists, had a law which punished the drinking of wine, with death, unless it was taken as a medicine prescribed by a physician. In Rome young people were not allowed to drink until their thirtieth year.

Many regulations of this kind or worse have existed in civilized countries at all times without being respected. By the capitularies of Charlemagne in 801, priests were prohibited from drinking or inducing others to drink.[9] Whoever disobeyed this law was to be excommunicated or corporally chastised,[10] for drink is the source of all evils. The same order was given to the army. In the year 812, a regulation was issued prohibiting soldiers from inducing others to drink, and if one of them were discovered in a state of drunkenness he was to be excommunicated and sentenced to live on water until he had repented of his evil behaviour. In spite of interdictions of this kind, reinforced by those of Church councils, drinking continued even in sacred places. This state of affairs went on, although there was no lack of attempts in the following centuries to alarm drinkers by terrifying pictures of alcoholic abuse and its consequences. In 1524, the Electors of Treves and the Palatinate, the five Counts Palatine of the Rhine, the margrave Casimir of Brandenburg, the landgrave of Hesse, the bishops of Würzburg, Strasbourg, Speyer, Regensburg, etc., founded a temperance society which not only bound them personally but also obliged them to proselytize. They also pledged themselves instantly to dismiss functionaries in their service who drank, and to note the cause of the dismissal on their certificates.

In France, in the reign of François I, an edict of the year 1536 stipulated that anyone who appeared in public in a state of intoxication should on the first occasion by imprisoned on bread and water, on the second chastised with birch and whip, and on the third publicly flogged. Should further relapses occur the delinquent was to have an ear cut off and suffer banishment. Exemption from punishment for infringement of the laws during the state of inebriety was quite out of the question. All these numerous and infinitely varied measures taken in recent centuries against alcoholism, like the modern forms of prohibition, have hardly ever achieved any appreciable result, for the reason already stated.

The latest methods[11] of dealing with the question, though conceived, it is true, with the best intentions, will be no more of a success, for they are for the most part the work of jurists. A knowledge of the technique of law-making is not sufficient to cope with problems of this kind. What the modern jurist has introduced into legislation, for instance the conception of the responsibility of the alcoholic, is inapplicable in practice. The conception of responsibility includes free will, foreknowledge of the consequences of an action. But this may be lacking after the use alcoholic beverages for two reasons.

(1) It is impossible for the drinker himself to foresee the limits of his individual resistance, i.e. the dangerous moment may be missed when the individual is still free from moral reproach after

imbibing a certain quantity, while if he drinks more he will become morally culpable and therefore worthy of condemnation.

(2) It is impossible for the drinker to estimate correctly in all cases the intoxicating strength of the beverage he is consuming.

When an individual is in a state of intoxication it is not circumstantially evident whether he has knowingly or unknowingly consumed methyl alcohol, fusel oil, nitrobenzine, disagreeable essential oils, or other ingredients contained in the beverage without which he would not have become drunk or committed a criminal offence.

If there is no culpability, there can be no penalty. The individual cannot be "morally reproached." In my opinion it is not possible to formulate a law applicable equally to the abuse of alcohol and the apparent consequences. Even the richest toxicological experience is bound to fail in seeking to prevent drunkenness. In the school and the home efforts must be made to prevent the development of alcoholism. Especially in the schools sufficient time must be devoted to teaching this part of the "science of life." Many other ideas bordering on this subject could at the same time be installed into the young brain and the growing intelligence.

LIQUOR HOFFMANNI

The pharmacopœia contains the formula of a mixture of three parts alcohol and one part ether. A large number of "abstainers," especially women, employ this spirit of ether as a remedy against states of depression from which they frequently suffer. They would protest at being called alcoholists or etheromaniacs. Nevertheless they are to a certain degree slaves to the habit, which often becomes a mania. I know a court case where a woman was said to have consumed within four years thirty thousand marks' worth of this liquid. Attention should be paid to drinkers of such draughts.

CHLOROFORM

Scarcely a year after the first application of chloroform as an anæsthetic there were already persons who habitually inhaled it in order to experience agreeable sensations. At that time many warnings were issued pointing out that this abuse was liable to give rise to acute and chronic mental diseases. The number of chloroform inhalers has since that time considerably increased, as I reported in 1893.[12] Physicians, pharmacists, hospital attendants, and druggists are among those who most frequently indulge in this passion. Some take the drug many times a day, some more rarely, and others at intervals of two to three days. Occasionally chloroform is inhaled like ether and taken internally. The habit creates a power of resistance, which, however, is very limited. The great majority of chloroformists fall ill after a more or less short lapse of time. The chloroform-free interval, however, is nearly always shorter than in the case of morphia. In one case chloroform had been inhaled against attacks of eclampsia, and later against headache and backache. The patient was irritable and soon began to crave for chloroform as if she had been using it for years. It was refused, and a typical mental disease with hallucinations, persecution-mania, etc., appeared. If an individual habituated to chloroform takes an excessive dose the consequences are just as serious as if one not accustomed to the drug had taken the same quantity. Perhaps the former succumb even more easily to the intoxication. For instance, a chemist's apprentice had acquired the habit of taking inhalations of chloroform every day on account of the excitation and agreeable sensations he experienced therefrom. One day, however, probably while still under the influence of the drug, he made a fresh inhalation and poured about 12 to 15 gr. of chloroform on a towel. He fell across the counter with his head on the towel and remained in this position for approximately ten minutes. When he was found his pulse had almost ceased to beat, and in spite of all conceivable efforts, it was impossible to recall him to life. The reasons leading to the use of chloroform are the same as for morphia.

Some morphinists indulge also in the abuse of chloroform. I once treated a colonel who, in order to break himself of the morphia habit, constantly sniffed at his handkerchief on which he had poured several drops of chloroform. The quantities consumed in twenty-four hours vary according to the degree of habituation and the violence of the craving for chloroform. It is nor rare for quantities of 40 to 360 gr., and in some cases probably more, to be inhaled daily. A pharmacist inhaled in this way 8,000 gr. of chloroform in two months. A morphinist in whom morphia did not induce sleep spent the greater part of the day in bed and chloroformed himself every time he awakened. Another began by pouring some drops of chloroform on a handkerchief held to his nose until his sense-impressions were diminished. At night he applied larger quantities. Later on the craving for the narcotic became so violent that he applied a small rag impregnated with chloroform almost the whole day long. All regard for his position and the entreaties of his relations vanished, and the quantity used in repeated doses amounted in volume to a ordinary wine bottleful in twenty-four hours, and at night alone 500 gr. The passionate desire for a new inhalation is in many cases just as powerful as the craving for morphia in inveterate morphinists.

Physical and mental troubles are the consequence of the mania for chloroform. Digestion suffers, epigastric pains and vomiting of the contents of the stomach and of blood occur occasionally after internal application of chloroform and even after inhalations. Physical weakness and emaciation are very apparent. In some cases jaundice occurs. I have seen the latter, for instance, in a physician who inhaled chloroform only every two or three days. The sexual impulse generally disappears. I consider a local irritation of the mucus of the nose, which incites the patient to incessant snuffling, a significant symptom for the diagnosis of this mania. Trembling of the limbs is frequently observed. General marasmus is usually the ultimate phenomenon of the intoxication.

In the great majority of cases disturbances of the central nervous system, especially of the mental state, occur. These may either come about periodically or be permanent. The subjects generally exhibit a marked deterioration in their moral conduct. They nearly always lie; their memory weakens, and the mental functions are retarded. Their character is suspicious, irresolute, capricious, and passes from one extreme to the other. They are irritable and extremely susceptible. They sleep little or not at all. In some cases neuralgic disorders set in, racking pains in the limbs, and sometimes lumbar pains also. Occasionally these patients experience hallucinations which may be succeeded by a state similar to delirium tremens with alcoholicum. Others are suddenly seized by attacks of mental derangement with persecution-mania. Some create the impression of dipsomaniacs. They usually appear quite normal; with the periodic appearance of a certain excitation they change. They demand chloroform eagerly and violently, and decay both physically and intellectually.

Some of these toxicomaniacs are obliged to spend the rest of their lives in asylums after a relatively short abuse of the drug, other after many relapses. The latter case is appropriately illustrated by a certain physician who became a chloroform addict in a very peculiar manner. His father, a medical man, himself suffered from heart disease and used to employ chloroform for his complaint until his death. The son, desirous of knowing whether chloroform inhalations had contributed to his father's death, experimented with the drug on himself. His subsequent experiences soon rendered its application indispensable. Two years later mental derangement with persecution-mania set in and brought him into an asylum. Temporary discontinuance of the narcotic brought no relief. He relapsed again and again and finally became a permanent asylum inmate. On the other hand, we have a striking example of how the effects of the drug can for a long time be resisted. For thirty years a woman employed the narcotic both by inhalation and internal application, also using ether and strong wine. When seventy years old she suffered from violent delirium so that she had to be tied down in bed. It was stated that after having been cured of a disease she ceased to take chloroform, but became addicted to liquor Hoffmanni and alcohol. Her intelligence and her memory do not seem to have been greatly affected.

This extreme variety in the symptoms is the result of the supreme influence of the personality. The wife of a physician was addicted to chloroform. In the presence of her husband she was operated on for a small abscess and inhaled chloroform until stupefied. She passed into a state of semi-narcosis resembling the rigidity of death. From that day forward she never returned to a normal state; her skin became discoloured, she grew emaciated, and died two years later. In all probability the abuse of the drug was clandestinely continued.

On the withdrawal of chloroform, symptoms similar to those of demorphinization generally appear. The excitation assumes quite unusual proportions. Under the influence of excessively terrifying illusions, and hallucinations of sight and hearing, the patients are seized with raving madness, break everything they can get hold of, incessantly throw themselves about, and scream until fatigue renders the continuance of their fury impossible. Vomiting, diarrhœa and cardiac weakness are apt to accompany the mental symptoms. In the case of a person with a psychopathic disposition who had for fifteen years inhaled 40 to 60 gr. chloroform spirit, equal to 20 to 30 gr. pure chloroform, daily, and had occasional attacks of delirium, symptoms of withdrawal were almost completely lacking. The possibility of a cure occurs when the use of the narcotic has not lasted too long, but even then it is not certain. Inveterate chloroform-inhalers are incurable. It is only very ignorant people who believe in the so-called "cures" in two and a half to five days.

Paragraph 51 of the German Penal Code has also been applied in the case of a chloroformist, aged twenty, accused of theft. He was acquitted because he had been addicted to the narcotic for five years, and when committing the deed was still under the influence of chloroform inebriety.

ETHER

What I have said in the preceding pages about the habitual use of narcotic remedies with respect to chloroform is also applicable to ether. Even forty-five to fifty years before the recommendation of ether for medicinal use it had been applied as a narcotic. From England etheromania penetrated into France, Germany, etc., without its devotees becoming very numerous in the two latter countries, for morphia soon appeared on the horizon, possessing some advantages over ether especially as regards to clandestine application. Unfortunately there are still many persons who make use of ether for their pleasure in the form of inhalations or by internal administration in increasing quantities.

The reasons which lead to this practice are very various. Among them are imitation, seduction exercised by the description of its agreeable effects, the alleviation of physical or mental troubles. Individual sensibility brings about great variety in the character of the effects. Illusions of sight and hearing, dreams of paradisal happiness in accordance with the desires of the person concerned, the hearing of pleasant music, visions of beautiful women and lascivious situations, and many other illusions may be experienced, enduring for some time and leaving behind them the remembrance of a wonderful dream. A French poet has referred to the impressions of a woman in child-bed under the influence of a narcosis as the acme of agreeable sensation which this substance is capable of evoking.

Oh, d'un double mystère ineffable pouvoir;
Au moment qu'elle enfante elle croit concevoir.

Habituation gives rise finally to the toleration of considerable doses, but does not prevent death if the inhalation is too prolonged. Ether-users are also liable to death from acute intoxication, especially if they do not eat regularly. Physical and mental disturbances appear after a more or less short lapse of time. Defects of moral conduct in particular are not slow to occur. The mania for ether has even seized the younger generation, although not to a great extent.

A ten-year-old boy who, with the exception of a slight noise in the first cardiac sound and an anæmic paleness, seemed to be in the best of health, was extremely intelligent and precocious and himself attributed his extraordinary successes at school to the use of ether. At the beginning he drank 20 to 50 gr. and even 100 gr. a day, and at night inhaled the same quantity in the form of vapour. After awakening from ether inebriety he was able to solve the most difficult mathematical problems. All attempts to cure him of this mania were futile. He stole money from his parents and broke into pharmacies in order to obtain the drug. In the course of nine years the quantity consumed daily increased to one litre, to which in the last year he added subcutaneous morphia injections. He died of heart failure which I attribute, according to my present experience, to the abuse of ether.

There are also persons who never take ether internally, but merely inhale its vapour in the manner of chloroform-inhalers. In a case of this kind the habitué, an educated man, showed signs of organic debility, and was in danger of losing his social position. He was tired and weak, had no appetite, suffered from muscular trembling, and exhaled a disagreeable odour. In another case an ether-inhaler indulged in the mania when driving in a carriage in order to conceal his addiction to the drug. He slowly inhaled the ether, thus prolonging the state of excitation, during which he quarrelled and fought with the coachman, frequently rendering police intervention necessary.

A woman whose father had been a drunkard and the mother a "nervous eccentric," had at the age of twenty-two taken ether for four months in increasing doses for medicinal purposes. She then ceased to take the drug but began again to employ ether at the age of forty-two for the same reasons. The need increased to such an extent that she applied approximately 250 gr. in the course of every night. Her organism suffered, she became emaciated, pale and anæmic, and complained of gastric pains. She was irritable and suspicious, had suicidal intentions, wandered about alone at night, and slept on public benches in a state of ether inebriety. Finally this patient, who had been a society lady, begged in the streets in order to be in a position to indulge in her passion. She is said to have been cured after withdrawal treatment.

The habit of drinking ether seems to be comparatively common. It is easy to understand that in those countries where anti-alcoholism has succeeded in attaining an outward victory, the craving for another inebriating substance leads to the discovery of substitutes. Ether is one of these succedanea. Not a drop of alcohol is taken, but ether and spirit of ether is used in increasing quantities. It is not considered as becoming in the female sex to consume large quantities of concentrated alcohol habitually, and for this reason women contribute a large contingent to etheromania. A small phial of ether is an indispensable vade-mecum for such women. Many drinkers of ether take excessive daily doses. For instance, the chemist Bucquet consumed over half a litre and Rouelle one litre daily.

The organic disturbances generally begin with disorders of the functions of the stomach. Dyspepsia, gastric pains, and vomiting set in. Trembling, muscular weakness, and glycosuria are less frequent. In the case of a woman who had consumed ether poured on sugar every day before meals and had in the course of two and a half months taken in all 180 gr., weakness and trembling of the hands and feet, morbid contraction of certain muscles of the legs when walking, pains in the thorax and between the shoulder-blades, vomiting, tinnitus aurium, headache, palpitation of the heart, and cramps in the calves appeared and the patient had no appetite. In the morning vomiting occurs as in the case of heavy drinkers. The activity of the heart soon becomes irregular and weak, the skin assumes a pallid hue. The character also soon changes. Irritability, sudden changes of temper, capriciousness and concurrent loss of will-power can be observed. The subjects are negligent and lazy. It has on the other hand been pointed out that delirium does not occur as with alcoholists, nor cachexia as with morphinists. It is said that among the Irish ether-drinkers, now to be described, there are some cases in which mental modification alone occurs and the physical state is not affected. It has even been considered a blessing that the Catholic clergy have persuaded the Irish to abandon alcohol in favour of the harmless ether.

For some time attention has been drawn to the fact that in Ireland the drinking of ether seems to be becoming very popular. The origin of this abuse has not been ascertained. It is stated on the one hand that the Irish peasants began ether-drinking in the year 1840, at the time of Father Mathew's preaching against alcohol, and on the other that medical men prescribed ether too liberally. The reason for this mischief has also been sought, however, in the limitation of the alcohol distilleries. The inhabitants of Northern Ireland drink the cheap ether manufactured in England mixed with alcohol. In Northern Ireland more ether is used than in the whole of England. On market days in Draperstown and Cookstown the air used to be filled with the vapour of ether, and the same odour impregnated the carriages of the local railway. In this part of the country, men, women, and children drink ether, the former doses of 8 to 15 gr. repeatedly one after the other. In order to alleviate the burning sensation which the drug produces and to reduce the loss by belching, the addicts drink water after the doses of the narcotic. Some of them can tolerate 150 to 500 gr. of ether in several portions. Intoxication sets in rapidly and disappears with the same speed. The initial symptoms consist in violent excitation, profuse salivation and eructation. Occasionally, convulsions similar to those of epilepsy occur. A state of stupor is evoked after the consumption of very large doses. Ether-drinkers of this kind are quarrelsome, tend to become liars, and suffer from gastric disorders and nervous prostration.

In consequence of these facts the retail sale of ether has been regulated. The drug is now included in the list of poisons, and is only supplied in pharmacies on production of a written authorization.

In Norway the use of ether seems to have assumed large proportions. On holidays old and young, men and women consume the drug.

In some German districts, especially in the neighbourhood of Memel and Heydekrug, the drinking of ether has assumed the form of an epidemic among the Lithuanian inhabitants. In 1897 in the town of Memel alone 69 carboys of 60 litres, and in the district of Memel 74 carboys of 70 litres, 8,580 litres in all, were sold for drinking purposes.

On market days the smell of ether exhaled by the drinkers is notice-able at every turn. When, on the road between Heydekrug and the neighbouring villages, a carriage with noisy inmates drawn by a madly galloping horse which the intoxicated driver is unmercifully beating, passes the wayfarer, a strong smell of ether can be ascertained in the rush of air.

When the market is closed many men and women intoxicated with ether can be seen reeling about. Even children are habituated to ether at a very delicate age. School children have suffered mentally to a large extent in consequence. Whole families have been ruined by habitual consumption of ether. I cannot say how far the state of affairs has changed since the war.

In Russia, and especially in Galicia, country doctors observed a similar epidemic. The poorer inhabitants of the country are particu-larly addicted to ether. Mixed with a small amount of alcohol it is consumed in inconceivable quantities. In these people a kind of mor-bid stupidity develops which in serious cases renders thought impos-sible. Cardiac disorders usually terminate their lives.

Particular cases prove that ether also has its victims in high soci-ety. In one case an English baronet used morphia and ether concur-rently for three years and succumbed to his passion. In another case an etheromaniac earl committed extravagances which, from a moral point of view, classified him among mental deficients.

I have no doubt that anatomical investigation of ether drinkers would show modifications similar to those of alcoholists.

A cure for this mania is all but impossible. Withdrawal has been accomplished, but it is only rarely that relapses do not set in. During treatment, deprivation symptoms occur as in morphinism. Insomnia is very marked, delirium occasionally occurs followed by convulsions. A patient has been known to succumb to the latter.

BENZINE

In some persons the evil habit of intentionally inhaling the vapours of benzine in order to experience agreeable sensations has been ascer-tained. That benzine should give rise to such effects is not surprising, for it belongs to the chloroform-ether group which has the property of modifying the chemical equilibrium of the constituents of the brain. I was the first to state[13] that all volatile substances capable of dissolving the fatty matter of the brain also exercise an influence on its functions, this latter action being proportionate to the dissolving capacity and being exercised even on the sensory nerves, for instance, the fibres of the optic nerves.

It is true that cases of benzinomania are comparatively rare; they are, however, interesting because they manifest the shifts to which men can be reduced in the desire to experience cerebral sensations different from those of everyday life. Petrol seems unsuitable for this purpose, but it is used, and its use continued if its effects are agreeable experiences.

Some children and adults who habitually inhaled petrol vapour for their pleasure have been the object of various investigations. A girl suffered from disagreeable disturbances of sight due to a central scotome. According to the report of her mother, who cleaned gloves for a living, she had had for some years the habit of smelling at a rag soaked in benzine or of holding the petrol bottle to her nose. Especially before bedtime the craving was so violent that neither punishment nor entreaty was of any avail, and although the mother attempted to lock up her store of benzine the patient had her own supply which she always replenished from a hiding place in the garden. The girl bought more of the liquid as soon as she had collected a few pence. She was removed from home and placed in a convent. According to the evidence of the nuns, she was not able to indulge in her old habit, although during the first few days she did everything she could to obtain petrol. After three months the relative scotome for red and green had completely disappeared, but normal sight which had been disturbed was not re-established.

Benzinomaniac glove-cleaners have also been observed. The statement of a man who used benzine in his business apprises us of the sensations experienced after the inhalation of the vapour. He declared that he had previously consumed a considerable amount of liquor, but for six months not a drop had passed his lips. He had inhaled petrol vapour instead, this being abundantly at his disposal in his profession as a bandage-maker, and these inhalations had been completely substituted for alcohol. He said he had experienced a wonderful feeling of peace, and agreeable delicious dreams. A colleague from southern Germany had taught him this way of applying petrol. But the agreeable effects of benzine diminished after some time. Hallucinations appeared, the patient heard the unpleasant music of barrel-organs and unharmonious singing by voices known to him; red ants crept about on his body, he saw several figures of animals and dwarfs, and once the whole room seemed to be full of coloured silk threads which fluttered to and fro.

In all probability these symptoms were due to the effects of benzine, and cannot be explained by the cessation of the use of alcohol.

NITROUS OXIDE

A chemist gradually acquired the habit of inhaling every day a small quantity of nitrous oxide (laughing gas). At the beginning the sweetish smell of the gas was very unpleasant, but he slowly became used to it. In order to be able to inhale the gas at all times he fitted a small apparatus to the reservoir from which he could easily take a whiff. This gave rise to a permanent state of inebriety, the source of extremely pleasant sensations. He had wonderful dreams in which he saw beautiful landscapes, marvelous figures and scenes. The young man soon began to neglect his duties, but could not renounce his passion. He went mad and ended in an asylum.

HYPNOTICA: SOPORIFICS

Insomnia is one of the worst evils from which mankind can suffer. It is always a calamity, whether the victim be a worker who during the day attends to his business or an idle pleasure-seeker. Woe to the unhappy wretch tortured by this evil who lies awake till morning on his hard or soft couch. But those too in whom mental overwork has excited the cerebral functions so that sleep refuses to come, or whose eyes will not close for fear of the coming morn, those whose unbalanced soul vibrates convulsively or whose conscience banishes sleep in self-accusation, all vainly look forward for many a long night to the realization of Egmont's words:

> Sweet sleep, thou comest like a pure joy of thine own accord, without supplication of prayer. Thou dissolvest the knots of grave thoughts, thou interweavest pictures of sorrow and of joy; the course of internal harmony flows without an obstacle, and lulled in agreeable frenzy we sink and cease to be.

And how often in the darkness of sleepless nights is not the sad and sighing complaint sounded unto eternity that sleep might favour those who hour after hour vainly expect the appearance of dawn? How grievous is the cry of Shakespeare's King Henry IV:

> *. . . O sleep, O gentle sleep,*
> *Nature's soft nurse, how have I frighted thee,*
> *That thou no more wilt weight my eyelids down*
> *And steep my senses in forgetfulness? . . .*
> *O thou dull god, why liest thou with the vile*
> *In loathsome beds, and leav'st the kingly couch*
> *A watch-case or a common 'larum-bell? . . .*
> *Canst thou, O partial sleep, give thy repose?*

Mental and physical fatigue finally demand aid at any price.

What remedies do we possess against the waves of restlessness of the brain? King Xerxes of old, when he could not sleep one night, had the chronicle of the empire read to him in order to become fatigued. His sleeplessness brought the highest royal honours to Mordechai, salvation to the Jews of the empire, and to Haman the gallows. It is unlikely that Xerxes slept that night! Sometimes indeed the reading of a very dull book is a remedy; medical books written by regular professors of the faculty are especially liable to produce sleep. As a rule, persons who suffer from insomnia have recourse not to mental remedies but to chemical substances.

The physical and mental consequences of the latter have been the subject of research which informs us that the satisfaction of the need for sleep by their means has in many cases led to a permanent craving for them. Those who use them can hardly wait for the evening in order to be transferred from the life of reality to that of dreams. It is, furthermore, certain that the toleration of a prolonged use of hypnotics depends upon the brain constitution of the individual, the chemical composition of the hypnotic, and the chemical relationship between the elements of the brain and the drug. The differences of toleration are under these circumstances very considerable. No devotee of sporific remedies remains immune, in the long run, from harmful effects. Even if these effects are felt scarcely or not at all, they are always present to a greater or lesser degree as the price paid for sleep, in the form of nervous disorders or other morbid states which result from abuse, and on examination do not fail to be discovered. In the following pages I describe some of the hypnotics which have become more popular and which are most frequently abused. The results of my observations may without restriction be extended to other substances used for the same purpose but not mentioned in this book.

Efforts to restrict the abuse of narcotic substances encounter a serious obstacle in the activities of certain manufacturers of chemical products who have at their disposal a whole staff of medical and even philological advisers. The propaganda litreature of these firms, which is constantly changed, and even written in Latin with quotations from Roman poets, endeavours to influence medical men and to cause them to prescribe the soporifics in question, which are always untruthfully declared to be non-poisonous or of a "considerable degree of nontoxicity."

The consequences are apt to be very serious if, thus disguised, danger-ous substances which powerfully influence the brain fall into the hands of persons suffering from insomnia who have once tasted the charm of sleep produced *ad libitum*, and would at all costs retain it. There is no hypnotic whose use is harmless, and medical men should take this to heart in order to prevent the increase of the already widespread evil of soporific consumption. Profiteering may flourish elsewhere, but in this sphere it is apt to give rise to injurious poison-blossoms.

CHLORAL

Many of the motives which lead to the application and abuse of mor-phia coincide with those which give rise to the employment of chlo-ral. Fortunately the latter is fairly rare, for chloral has virtually been erased from the list of medicaments; it is unpleasant to take, and the injurious consequences of its habitual use are too well known. Soon after its introduction into therapeutics the avarice of traders and oth-ers interested in its application produced many chloralists. Many of these applaud the harmlessness of the drug even after prolonged ap-plication; they are like the drunkard who glorifies alcohol as the source of all delights. A tendency exists to become habituated to chloral, as with every other narcotic substance. In some cases habituation and increase of the dose do not take place so rapidly as with morphia. There are, however, many proofs that such persons have a passionate craving for chloral, i.e. that the substance has taken the place of a normal excitant. There is no doubt that chloral is far more dangerous than morphia in this respect, not only because it is liable to call forth serious disturbances in the central organs, but also because there is the possibility of sudden death from paralysis of the heart. In many cases of sudden death this real cause is not diagnosed. The doses con-sumed daily amount in some cases to 15–20 gr. The combination of chloral with morphia also occurs. The following description depicts the effects of chloral.

In some chloralists the face becomes very red, almost purple; others exhibit a lurid discoloured appearance soon after ingestion of the sub-stance. The eyeballs frequently grow yellowish, the skin is covered with spots, blood-spots, papular eruptions, etc. The fingers are ulcerated and the finger-nails spoilt. The general condition of health suffers. A feeling of intense cold, fatigue, and faintness, is accompanied by gastro-intestinal disorders, indigestion, and a considerable degree of emaciation. Habitual use is also said to occasion spasms of the bladder and other urinary troubles, weakness and palpitation of the heart, respiratory disturbances, pneumonia, and occasionally gangrene from pressure. The sexual impulse is generally lacking and troubles of menstruation occur. In addition to these symptoms, pains in the limbs, often also in the back and in the joints, increased cutaneous sensibility, formication, weakness of the legs, facial paralysis, etc., frequently appear in some combination or other.

Chloralists are, like morphinists, morally weak and incapable of renouncing their passion. Their insomnia is often increased by abuse of the narcotic. The mental faculties are enfeebled so that the behavior of some of them is childish and stupid. Their memory is affected, and in the advanced stages they become mentally and physically unfit. In many cases an exaggerated nervousness appears in the foreground. The patient is a prey to an incessant haste and restlessness which prevents him from staying in the same place even for a moment. From this state to real mental disease is only a step. In chloralists a state of raving madness, delirium and hallucination, have been observed. Morbid states of melancholia together with prostration, general weakness, cachectic appearance, refusal to take food, and suicidal intentions occur. The mental disposition of the subjects grows more and more sombre and they became misanthropes. Suicides as a result of chloralism are probably more frequent than has been assumed. They must be directly attributed to chloral since it creates a false mental disposition. A chloralist once attempted suicide with an excessive dose of chloral. He was cured from the acute symptoms, but remained an idiot.

Among the motor disturbances due to chloral, trembling of the hands and the head, ataxic walking, epileptoid convulsions with or without mental derangement may be observed. Convulsions with unconsciousness frequently occurred in a devotee of morphia and chloral. Between the crises he remained in a state of sleep from which he could be awakened. If the application of chloral was suspended unconsciousness disappeared, but weakness of memory and temporary mental confusion remained. Another often had hallucinations and was always in a state of mental depression. One day he fell down in an epileptic fit.

The mental disease with which Nietzsche was affected is attributed to the hyper-productivity of his brain and to the continually increasing rapidity of his thinking as well as the use of chloral. I consider the latter circumstance particularly aggravating. His mind was so incessantly active that he found no sleep at night. Physicians recommended chloral for the foolish reason that this product is quite harmless. He took immediate doses of the drug, and in this way at least accelerated his mental ruin.

Gutzkow became a slave of the drug in the same manner, for he suffered from obstinate insomnia. One night in December, 1878, after having taken a dose of chloral he upset the light in a state of torpor and set fire to his bed. He never awoke again.

The cure of chloralism is attempted in the same manner as in morphinism, has the same consequences, and as regards success is just as futile as the latter. The gradual or rapid withdrawal of the drug, with or without the administration of small doses of morphia, always shows the severity of the detrimental effects which chloral has had on the economy of the organism, especially the brain. Generally violent excitation, excessive restlessness, states of fury, and raving with hallucinatory madness on a foundation of extreme depression occur. In one case the patient was almost exclusively tormented with hallucinations of hearing. In spite of the administration of morphia and alcohol in another patient, four days after deprivation extreme agitation and a mania for destruction occurred together with hallucinations of sight which lasted forty-eight hours. Trembling continued after the disappearance of the hallucinations. Complete retrogression of these states of excitation may take place after a few days, or sometimes not till weeks have passed. Pains and twitching in the legs, especially the thighs and the calves, weakness and alternating frequency of the pulse, attacks of cardiac weakness, diarrhœa, twitching of the facial muscles, trembling of the tongue, stammering speech are more frequent symptoms.

Veronal

This substance may also become the object of habitual use which is not rarely accompanied by a progressive increase in the size of the doses. Like all toxins that act on the brain, it produces a euphoric state. A morphinist had for two months taken 4 gr. of veronal per day, i.e. 250 gr. in all. This sufficed to call forth motor incoordination, weakness, tottering gait, drawling, muttering speech, and on the mental side a stimulation of the imagination and a state of euphoric gaiety as in inebriety. In those cases where the abuse has been more prolonged the symptoms are far more serious. The individual sensibility of different subjects to veronal plays an extremely important part in deciding the form of the disturbances of the organic functions produced by the drug. These troubles appear even if the daily dose does not exceed 0.5 gr. If the subject is very sensitive, disorders of metabolism, rapid emaciation, hæmatic disturbances will soon be observed. In the blood an unpleasant decomposition-product of the colouring matter, hæmatoporphyrin, is formed, which passes into the urine. In one case veronal gave rise to these symptoms after six months' use.

Certain nervous persons who suffer from insomnia experience an urgent desire for a further application of the drug even if the initial doses medically prescribed already give rise to alarm signals in the form of drowsiness in the daytime, motor disturbances, etc. A young hysterical girl considered these symptoms as negligible and procured veronal on old prescriptions which finally she took in daily doses of 1 to 2 gr. for eleven and a half months. She spent seven months in bed with progressive loss of strength and nausea. She suffered from extreme excitation, slight confusional illusions, defects of memory, and tottering gait. After admission to a hospital more serious disturbances of consciousness occurred, interrupted by lucid intervals, and after eleven days unilateral twitching of the face, immobility of the pupil, and general convulsions supervened. She died during an attack of these convulsions. Disease and death were without doubt due to veronalism.

I do not think that veronalists are rare.

PARALDEHYDE

The inclination of many persons to take narcotics renders the abuse of paraldehyde quite natural. Patients have been observed who took 35 to 40 gr. of the substance per day, sometimes even more. One of them continued the abuse for over a year. A man has been known to reach in the course of twenty-six months a weekly dose of 480 gr. The symptoms produced are similar to those of chronic alcoholism: emaciation and anæmia, fever in the evening, constipation and flatulence accompanied by voracity, irregular activity of the heart and palpitations, albuminuria, hallucinations of hearing and sight with illusions or delirium tremens, defects of memory and intelligence, disturbances of speech, a feeling of stupor or anxiety and excitement, muscular weakness, trembling of the tongue, face and hands, uncertain gait, restlessness, and paræsthesia. In spite of cautious withdrawal, deliria with convulsions similar to epilepsy are apt to occur. A lady, who after using morphia and chloral had become addicted to paraldehyde and was unable to sleep without the substance, became agitated, depressed, suffered neuralgic pains, and collapsed if deprivation of the drug only lasted for a few hours. Menstruation had ceased and a cure was impossible.

SULPHONAL

After reading the preceding pages it will not seem surprising that man has become addicted to this substance also and finds pleasure in its use. Its abuse inevitably produces organic modifications, especially alterations in the blood, where hæmatoporphyrin is formed from oxyhæmoglobin. Symptoms of paralysis of the limbs and trunk have also been ascertained, and in the intellectual sphere, weakness of memory, somnolence, disorders of speech, etc. A withdrawal cure after three to five months' abuse produced faintness and motor disturbances.

POTASSIUM BROMIDE

On account of the cheapness of potassium bromide and the facility with which it can be procured, the over-worked who suffer from insomnia make use of it and soon become slaves to it, as does the morphinist to morphia.[1] Indeed many persons lie with respect to its use, in the same way as morphinists, and positive proofs are frequently necessary to obtain a confession. Abuse increases with use, so that various disorders of health occur. The substance does not, however, produce a euphoric state.

The bromide salt spreads throughout the organism. The brain retains considerable amounts. If a woman employs the drug before or during pregnancy her child is apt to suffer from bromine poisoning. A newly-born child of this description was emaciated, the skin hung loosely like an empty sack round the thighs, the face had a senile appearance and was of a bluish colour. The infant slept incessantly and only awaked in the morning and at night for a few short moments. Later on grave dermatitis occurred similar to that which frequently affects consumers of bromides, and which is apt to develop into nodulous and ulcerous formations.

The limits of individual sensibility are very wide here also. Habituation to bromides gradually produces an attenuation of their action. The symptoms of habitual use are frequently the following: reduction of the sexual impulse, troubles of the respiratory and cardiac apparatus, a peculiar fixed expressionless stare, and especially disturbances of the functions of the brain, such as apathy, weakness of memory and understanding, etc. This mental depression is often accompanied by motor weakness and disturbances of co-ordination. Occasionally a state of excitation appears instead of depression. Unpleasant consequences are also liable to occur after deprivation.

Bromural

Habituation to this substance may likewise be induced by gradually increasing the dosage. The symptoms observed are disorders of speech and of the reflexes, interference with temporal and spatial perception, and insecure gait.

KAVA-KAVA

The immense island world of the Pacific attracts the attention of the anthropologist perhaps to a greater degree than the continental territories. For it leads us among other things to ask the following questions. Has nature in her marvellous creativeness endowed man with some narcotic plant whose effects may be agreeably experienced? Have the inhabitants of these distant islands surrounded by the mighty ocean, who lead so bare an existence on their small fragment of the earth, been instinctively led to the discovery of substances capable of raising even them above the daily monotony of a crude existence and supplying

sensations of a wholly different state of well-being? The existence and
use on these islands of *piper methysticum*, which I was the first to investigate,[2] answer these questions in the affirmative. I also found
confirmation of a fact to which I have repeatedly alluded when speaking of the development of the use of such substances: namely, that
there is no obstacle which can arrest the spread of a narcotic, not
even the sea with its menacing dangers for the natives of these islands. Not men alone, but the ocean itself yields to the power of narcotics. Kava-Kava or *piper methysticum* is characteristic of Oceania,
i.e. all those intertropical swarms of islands which are spread over an
area of 66 million square kilometres. Who taught the natives to employ the plant in the manner in which they use it, which is the best
possible way? An insoluble problem, like many others in this sphere.

Piper methysticum is a carefully cultivated piperaceous plant with
several varieties. It is called *kava, kava-kava, ava,* or *yangona*. It may
be found at an altitude of 500 to 304 metres above sea-level and is a
picturesque, shrub-like plant which grows in thick bushes. The character of its slow growth is similar to that of bamboo.

The most important part of the plant is the root. It is knotty, thick,
and provided with sarmentous radicles up to 1.8 metres in length,
which are sometimes threadlike in their extremities. When fresh it is
greyish-green, in a dried state greyish-brown, and weighs between 1
and 2 kilogrammes in the fresh state. After removal of the bark a
network of ligneous formation appears, partly filled with a soft and
yellowish cellular substance. The section of the fresh plant is yellow-
ish-white, greyish-white, lemon-coloured or pink, according to the
variety. The central part of the root is soft with a few ligneous bundles.
The substance contained in the ligneous bundles is soft, spongy, and
can easily be scratched out with the finger-nail.

Where and how Kava-Kava is drunk

In the Australian Archipelago, which extends over nearly 20 degrees
of latitude, live two groups of aborigines. The former, the Melanesians
or Papuans, have dark skin and woolly hair. They inhabit the area
bounded on the north by New Guinea, the Louisiade Archipelago,
the Solomon Islands, the New-Britain Archipelago, to which New
Caledonia and the Loyalty Islands in the south are attached; on the
east by the New Hebrides, the St. Cruz Islands, the Fiji group, and far

to the south, New Zealand, whose population, however, does not belong to this group. The second ethnical group is that of the Polynesians and Micronesians, with light-coloured skin and lank hair. They inhabit the outer girdle of the islands above mentioned, and the others scattered in the Pacific, the Caroline Islands, the Marianne, Gilbert, Samoa, Tonga, and Marquesas Islands, the Society Islands, the Fortunate Islands, the Hervey, the Austral, and the Paumotu Islands. The existence and use of kava-kava is said to be confined to the islands inhabited by the light-coloured aborigines, and not to occur at all in the group inhabited by Papuasians. Such a division cannot be accepted, for the use of kava-kava in New Guinea, which is mainly populated by Papuans, is beyond question, whereas its existence has not been proved on the Tokelau Islands and others whose natives are light-skinned.

My investigations as to the geographical extension of *piper methysticum* and its use have led to the following results:

It occurs in New Guinea. Miklouho-Maclay once sent me a report on an inebriating beverage, *keu,* which all the male inhabitants prepared from *piper methysticum* on festive occasions. Its use, however, was only permitted to persons of a certain age. This custom exists not only on the Maclay Coast, Astrolabe Bay, and Finch Bay, but also on the Fly River, and probably extends far to the east and north. In the Carolines many plantations of the plant have been destroyed by the missionaries, and the use of kava-kava has greatly diminished. It still exists, however, in the Solomon Islands. The plant grows in New Caledonia but is not used there. In the New Hebrides the consumption of kava-kava is practised beside that of betel. Kava-kava is drunk on Tanno, Erromango and Meli, and farther to the east in Rotuma and the Futuna Islands. The Fiji Islanders use it, and the natives of the Tonga Islands take it every morning. Girls crush the root between stones. On Samoa it is consumed in moderation. It is cultivated there in such amounts that it is exported. In 1908 34,350 kilos, and in 1909, although an earthquake had destroyed a part of the plantations, 16,299 kilos, were exported. On Wallis (Uvea), where an excellent variety of the plant occurs, the missionaries have abolished its use. It also occurs in the Cook Archipelago and in the Tubuai Islands. In the Society Islands the plant was cultivated in Cook's time (1768). At the present day the cultivation of the plant on Tahiti has completely ceased. Even in the year 1830 it was hardly possible to procure a single specimen. Some natives do not even know its name. In the interior of Tahiti, sporadic specimens, stunted and with poor stems, have been observed, as well as on Raiatea and Moorea. Kava-Kava also occurs in the Tuamotu Islands and the Marquesas Archipelago. In the latter it is cultivated and employed a great deal. It occurs in nearly all the eleven islands which this group comprises.

There are still kava-kava plantations on the Sandwich Islands. It seems, however, that the dissemination and use of the plant have given way in favour of alcoholic beverages.

The geographical boundaries of the occurrence and use of kava are therefore with a few exceptions confined to the islands in the intertropical zone, from 23° north latitude to 23° south latitude and from 135° east longitude to 130° west longitude.

Preparation and Use of Kava-Kava

Kava was intimately interwoven with the social, religious, and political life of the South Sea Islanders. It accompanied them on all their peaceful and war-like enterprises, whether in common or individual, and played a prominent part in all the joyous or sad events of life. It is therefore not surprising that the first explorers of those islands spoke in detail of the plant and its use. Moreover the sorcerers and medicine-men among the natives highly valued kava because it acts very rapidly after ingestion not only as a euphoric but also as an anodyne.

The missionaries did all they could to suppress the use of kava, probably not to the benefit of the natives. The violent campaign against kava by the Presbyterian missionaries cannot be justified in the least. It bears witness to the gross ignorance of the missionaries, who have made many a mistake elsewhere. Reason, hide thy face! The Anglican mission was less hostile to kava. There is no doubt whatever, that the physical and moral state of the natives has been, and is, far more damaged by the use of alcohol than by the consumption of kava. The missions are right in pointing out that crime and misery appeared in Tahiti together with the spread of drunkenness. The substitution for the use of kava of the almighty alcohol had already begun at the opening of the last century. The natives acquired a knowledge of the preparation of alcohol from fermented sugar-containing material which has given rise locally to the use of indigenous products of this kind. On the Marquesas Islands, for instance, spirits are obtained from fermented coco-nut milk.

Before the arrival of the missionaries the kava plantation was divided into three parts. The first and best was reserved for the evil gods; it was taboo, i.e. sacrosanct. The second was reserved for the Atu, the gods of sleep, and the third belonged to the family. Here also, as with many other narcotic substances which I have described, an intimate connection with religious conceptions may be observed. At the present day the part reserved for the gods has generally been abolished. In Samoa and the Wallis Islands alone some families still consecrate a few feet of land to the old gods. On some of the last-mentioned islands, however, there are kava fields which belong to the community and in which every family has a share.

The drinking of kava often takes place to celebrate a festival. The planting of trees, for instance, is celebrated by a kava feast. Kava is consumed when palavering with other tribes, during the discussion of public affairs, in society, and when entertaining guests in order to experience agreeable sensations. It is also used as a sedative medicament to give repose to the diseased or fatigued organism. In some islands it is consumed as a daily beverage, like our tea or coffee. On some of the scattered islands of the Pacific Ocean the natives receive Europeans and wait upon them with kava. Cook saw the natives drink the drug several times during the morning. The Samoans always take kava before meals and never after, and some of the elder folk drink a cup of the beverage before breakfast. Occasionally, kava feasts take place at night by the light of torches. In Wailevu these festivals were customary in honor of the foreigners. Some ardent kava-drinkers imbibe the beverage six to eight times a day. There are many Europeans living on these islands who frequently make use of the drug. The inferior classes of whites on the Fiji Islands must be counted among those. In good society it is considered as a sign of respectability to refrain from using kava.

In the New Hebrides there are said to exist public-houses for kava orgies, generally situated near a banana tree. At sunrise the men repair to these places for a cup of kava. In the Samoa Islands a public square in the neighbourhood of a banana tree serves for the same purpose. In other islands perhaps any hut is chosen with this end in view. The ceremonies which accompany the preparation and drinking of kava differ in the various groups of islands, and are sometimes even dissimilar in different districts of one and the same island. For instance, in the mountainous parts of the Fiji Islands the tune of the *meke* chants sung when brewing yangona and the movements of the bodies of the singers as they accompany their airs are quite different from those customary on the coast. In some parts the ceremonies are the same as in ancient times. In other places the levelling influence of civilization which has invaded these islands has only allowed the pleasure of drinking to be retained. The ceremonies have been shortened or abolished. The Samoans at public kava feasts pray to the gods for health, long life, a good harvest, and success in war. Generally women are not present at these feasts. However, in Samoa and other islands both women and men have been seen to participate. In Waja (to the west of Viti Levu) the women are said to have their own kava societies, similar to those on Tonga.

Old or young roots are cleaned and cut into suitable pieces after the bark has been removed. The root is then masticated. This method, which is the most general, is the primitive Tonga method, whereas the crushing of the root between stones, the Fiji method, is hardly in use. The individuals chosen for the process of mastication first clean their hands and their mouths. Usually they are young men and boys with good teeth, but the females also assist. On the Fiji Islands when a kava feast without ceremonies is celebrated, the root is masticated by girls who serve it while singing. Solemnly and slowly the root is chewed until the substance is fine and fibrous. It is not permitted to swallow any of the juice, which accumulates in the mouth.

The method employed in these islands by many whites and half-breeds, which consists in scraping the root on a grater without mastication and chewing it or merely macerating it with water, is said not to furnish a beverage of such good quality. It is even said that an infusion of scraped kava in water and masticated kava are as dissimilar in their effects as currant wine and champagne. Two mouthfuls of the substance generally suffice for one person. As soon as mastication is accomplished, the chewed lumps are placed in a wooden bowl made in one piece, which holds from 2 to 6 litres, and sufficient water is added. The man in charge of the bowl then stirs the liquid with his hands for a few minutes. From the moment that the water is poured into the bowl the ceremonial commences. This differs on the various islands and has not yet been completely abandoned. There is a solemn appeal to the gods, the departed spirits, etc. The extracted vegetable residue is removed after the water has been in contact with the masticated kava for a sufficient time. Each native has his own receptacle, usually the half of an empty coconut, which is filled with the prepared kava beverage and drunk to the accompaniment of special rites.

In appearance kava resembles an infusion of coffee with milk. It is of a dirty greyish-brown or greyish-white colour, especially when stirred, by reason of the fine greyish-yellow detritus of the root, which is not removed by the process of filtration practised by the natives. If little of this residue is present, or if the islanders pour the kava into their vessels after allowing it to settle, the liquid has a light or dark brown colour. The taste differs with the mode of preparation. It may be insipid or very bitter, aromatic or biting, soapy or astringent. The reason for the difference in taste lies in the degree of accuracy with which the insoluble residue of the root is separated from the fluid. The latter contains only a very small amount of the active and sapid substances in solution. The presence of resin is of the greatest importance. The more resin there is, the most intensive the taste. The natives do not seem to grow accustomed to the peculiar taste of the beverage, for Cook saw them grimace as they took it and afterwards shake themselves.

The Active Substances of Kava and their Action

Until my own researches began, it was generally assumed that the secret of the action of kava lay in its mode of preparation. It was said that during mastication the saliva transformed the starch of the root into sugar, and that this by fermentation turned into alcohol. I have proved this opinion false in every respect. This has not prevented several writers in their ignorance from reproducing this nonsense at a later date.

The only active principle of kava is a resinous substance which is found in the root accompanied by the crystalline and non-active *methysticin (Kavalin)*, that is ψ- methysticin, a substance which I called *yangonin* (the crystalline anhydrous methylic ester of yangona acid) and a lactone with the formula $C_{15}H_{14}O_4$. By a special process I have been enabled to split this resin up into two components, α- and β-kava-resin, of which the former had a more powerful action on the human body. The α-resin has the property, like cocaine, of anæsthetizing the mucous membranes and also the eye. Otherwise both resins are similar in action. A carefully prepared kava beverage taken in small quantity occasioned only slight and agreeable modifications of sensibility. In this form it is a stimulating beverage after the imbibition whereof hardships can be endured more easily. It refreshes the fatigued body and brightens and sharpens the intellectual faculties. Appetite is augmented, especially if it is taken half an hour before meals. Some travellers prefer it to champagne, but believe that its effects are only fully experienced in hot climates. If enough of the active principle is ingested peculiar narcotic phenomena appear. In the first report of Cook's travels it is stated that some of the crew had drunk of the beverage, and that effects were observed similar to those of a large dose of a spirituous liquor or of opium.

After doses that are not too strong a state of happy carelessness, content, and well-being appears without any physical or mental excitation. It is a real euphoric state which is accompanied by an increased muscular efficiency. At the beginning speech is fluent and lively and the hearing becomes more sensible to subtle impressions. Kava has a soothing effect. Those who drink it are never choleric, angry, aggressive and noisy, as in the case of alcohol. Both natives and whites look upon it as a sedative in case of accidents. Reason and consciousness remain unaffected. After the consumption of greater quantities, however, the limbs become weary, the muscles seem to be out of control of the will, the gait is slow and unsteady, and the subject appears half drunk. An urgent desire to lie down manifests itself. The eye sees objects before it but is unable to identify them with exactness. In the same way the ears hear everything, but the individual is unable to account for what he hears. Everything becomes more and more diffuse. The drinker succumbs to fatigue, and experiences a desire to sleep which is stronger than all other impressions. He becomes somnolent and finally falls asleep. Many Europeans have themselves experienced this action of kava which paralyses the senses like magic and finally leads to deep sleep. Frequently a state of somnolent torpor accompanied by incoherent dreams and occasionally erotic visions remains without sleep supervening.

The sleep is similar to that produced by alcohol, out of which the individual can be awakened only with difficulty. If moderate quantities have been consumed it occurs twenty to thirty minutes later, and lasts from two to eight hours according to the degree of habituation of the subject. If the beverage is concentrated, i.e. contains a large amount of the resinous components of kava, intoxication comes on much more rapidly. The drinkers are found lying in the very places where they have been drinking. Occasionally a short state of nervous trembling occurs before they fall asleep. No excitation precedes these symptoms.

The strongest kava is prepared in Rotuma. The natives amuse themselves by intoxicating the sailors who come on shore to such a degree that they are unable to stand or walk and have to be carried on board.

It will be readily understood that Europeans who have had the opportunity of experiencing the agreeable effects of kava, frequently make use of the beverage. Many reports certify that even educated Europeans can only with difficulty break off the habit of regular kava-drinking after they have found pleasure in its consumption. Many whites in a socially inferior position may be seen in the Fiji Islands in a state of kava inebriety. No injurious consequences of any importance have been established.

As regards its moral influence on the subject, this mania is like all other passions of a similar nature, morphinism, alcoholism, etc. The kava-drinker is incessantly tormented with the craving for his favourite beverage, which he cannot prepare for himself. It is a repugnant spectacle to see old and white-haired people, degenerate through prolonged abuse of the drug, going from house to house in order to beg for freshly prepared kava and often meeting with a refusal. Mental weakness has also been stated to follow from kavaism. It is said that old kava habitués have red, inflamed, bloodshot eyes, dull, bleary, and diminished in their functions. They become extremely emaciated, their hands tremble, and finally they cannot lift the drinking vessel to their mouths. Numerous cutaneous diseases of the natives of the South Seas, especially a kind of scaly eruption which results in a parchment-like state of the skin, have been attributed to the abuse of kava. I do not, however, consider it probable that kava is the original cause of these affections.

KANNA

Under the name of kanna (channa), Kolbe more than 200 years ago designated a plant whose root he found used by the Hottentots as a

means of enjoyment. They chewed it and kept it in their mouths for
some time, thus becoming excited and intoxicated. "Their animal
spirits were awakened, their eyes sparkled and their faces manifested
laughter and gaiety. Thousands of delightsome ideas appeared, and a
pleasant jollity which enabled them to be amused by the simplest jests.
By taking the substance to excess they lost consciousness and fell into
terrible delirium."

At the present day the name channa designates certain species of
mesembryanthemum, for instance M. *expansum* and M. *tortuosum*
(kaugoed), which occur in the hinterland of the Cape of Good Hope,
especially on the dry Karroo plateau, and also in Namaqualand, etc.
The root, leaves, and trunk of these mesembryanthema are crushed
and the resulting material chewed and smoked. M*esembryanthemum
tortuosum* contains an alkaloid with a sedative action, a vegetable substance which in frogs gives rise to paralysis and the arrest of respiration, and in rabbits to convulsions. It is said that 5 gr. of the drug
produce a state of torpor in man.

It is impossible that these plants should produce the phenomena
which Kolbe attributed to kanna. He probably confused their effects
with those of Indian hemp, to which the Hottentots are passionately
addicted. The results experimentally achieved reveal pharmacological properties of such little importance that it is inconceivable why
the Hottentots should have used the plant. We are confronted with a
gap in our knowledge which for the present cannot be filled. There
are other plants in those countries, for instance *sclerocarya caffra* and
sclerocarya schweinfurthi, which have an intoxicating action and are
used for this purpose.

EXCITANTIA

CHARACTER OF EXCITANTS

Certain very marked characteristics distinguish the substances belonging to the group of excitants from all the other drugs described in the preceding pages. Their action, which extends to the brain and particularly to the cerebral cortex, is a purely exciting or stimulating one, which, even if highly concentrated and intense, produces these effects without calling forth serious symptoms of fatigue or inhibition of the functions. In consequence the mental functions are maintained at their initial level for a longer period, in spite of the natural tendency to fatigue which is the result of all labour continued for some time. The sense-activity of the brain is also augmented by the use of several of these substances and this results in a more vivid perception of mental impressions. The will finds the central nervous system more obedient to its orders even with respect to muscular activity, which, however, is not subjectively felt as a constraint produced by the drug. In this respect, the action of the excitants differs from that of other substances. The consciousness of the subject is in no way diminished, his physical and intellectual work is executed with absolute freedom, at any rate provided that he does not employ the drug in unreasonable doses. Such quantities damage the functions of the brain and the others that depend thereon, by their excessive activity and give rise to disturbances due to morbid excitation.

Nearly all the substances belonging to this series exercise also a stimulating action on the heart. This property is of great value in medicine as a means of increasing the output of this organ in certain cases of cardiac diseases.

The use of several of these excitants has become a habit among both civilized and uncivilized races. From pole to pole, mankind is addicted to their use without distinction of religion or social status. From the moment when tobacco excited the astonishment of the first explorers of America, a few centuries were enough for it to enslave the whole world.

The amount of excitants used throughout the world is much greater than the sum of all the other substances applied to similar purposes. At the present day they play a very important part in economic life. They have lost their former character as unimportant phenomena and have become substances of great importance for many hundreds of millions of people, even indispensable necessities of life. They close the vast circle of substances which act on the brain, and perhaps more than other drugs they propound problems for science with respect to the mechanism of their effects on the cerebral activity, the point of access of their influence and the fundamental difference which, though they are cerebral excitants like the rest, characterises their action. To the physiology of the brain and to psychology, they present problems towards the solution of which hardly a step has yet been taken. We can perceive the biological effects of their action, but in vain do we inquire how the effects are produced.

CAMPHOR

When St. Hidegarde, the abbess of Ruprechtsberg, near Bingen, spoke of camphor in the twelfth century or when Petrus Magrus mentioned it about the year 1000 in his "Ricettario" and on the basis of his own observations, the origin and therapeutic properties of this substance had already been known in the Far East since the sixth century.

It is not known whether camphor was used at that time, or later, with the sole object of experiencing agreeable sensations. The fact that it was sent as an extremely costly tribute from the people to kings and princes, and by them to their fellows, does not seem to prove that this was the case. Between 1342 and 1352 the Emperor of China presented Pope Benedict XII with camphor, cotton, and precious stones.

The use of camphor as an agreeable cerebral excitant began on a small scale in our times, probably because the results of self-administration of the drug which led to its repeated use became public, or perhaps because the use made of the substance in South America, as a preventive of fever and in cholera epidemics, had not been forgotten.

For about twenty years there have been in the upper classes of English society, male and female camphor-eaters who take the substance either in milk, alcohol, or in the form of pills, etc. The like habit of taking the drug may be observed in the United States and in Slovakia. Women assert that it freshens the complexion, but the real reason for its employment seems to be the desire to experience a certain degree of excitation and inebriety. But I consider a special disposition for the drug indispensable.

After ingestion of 1.2 gr. the following symptoms may be ascertained: an agreeable warmth of the skin with general excitation of the nerves, an impulse to move, a tickling of the skin, and a peculiar ecstatic mental excitation similar to inebriety. One addict declared that "he saw his destiny full of magnificent possibilities clearly and distinctly before his very eyes." This state continued for one and a half hours. After ingestion of 2.4 gr. an urgent desire to move appeared. All movements were greatly facilitated, and when walking the limbs were lifted far more than necessary. Intellectual work was rendered impossible. A flood of thoughts appeared, ideas chased each other with great rapidity without any one being analysed. The subject lost consciousness of his personality. After vomiting consciousness returned, although distraction, forgetfulness, and vacancy of mind remained. On awaking, the state of intoxication seemed to have been extraordinarily long and full of events of which the subject did not remember one. After three hours he was able to pull himself together and return to full consciousness, but the disorder of the brain was so powerful that unconsciousness and convulsive movements set in again after one hour. This lasted another half-hour, after which the patient gradually regained his full perceptive faculties and a normal condition of the muscles.

Loss of the sense of location and short gaps in the memory usually succeed the gastric irritations and convulsions due to the action of camphor habitually taken. The lost memories finally reappear, but in a very peculiar manner, so that, according to the statement of an addict, all affairs, events, and things he had forgotten seemed new, as if he had had no previous knowledge of them. And, even after having recognized all the members of his family, the objects in his room seemed very strange and new, as if they had just been given to him.

In Slovakia, states of convulsion similar to epilepsy are so frequent in consumers of camphor that in this region all local cases of similar fits are directly attributed to the drug. It may therefore be classified among the series of those essential oils which exercise a powerfully exciting action on the central nervous system. Though it is true that it has the property of temporarily disturbing the intellectual faculties, I think it improbable that in the sum of the effects of camphor a state of well-being or euphory occurs.

BETEL

The craving of the betel-nut chewer[1] for his drug is hardly less strong than that of other drug-addicts for their respective intoxicants. With regard to the daily frequency and persistence with which betel is chewed, it even surpasses all other substances of the same kind. No product of the Far East is craved for with the same ardour as betel. The Siamese and Manilese would rather give up rice, the main support of their lives, than betel, which exercises a more imperative power on its habitués than does tobacco on smokers. To cease to chew betel is for a betel-chewer the same thing as dying. The greatest privations and sufferings of human life, insufficient or bad nourishment, hard work, rough weather, and illness lose their disagreeable character before the comforting action of betel. However, it is not only in the force of the desire which it inspires and the frequency with which it is used that betel surpasses the extent of the practice of chewing betel in the inhabited world, and the huge amounts consumed, give it a supreme position among all similar substances. Its use extends over 100° of longitude and about 20° of latitude. It can be found in nearly all countries between 68° and 178° east longitude, and between 12° south and 30° north latitude, over a territory of about eight million square kilometres comprising the huge area of the China Sea and the Indian and Pacific Oceans. From the Queen Charlotte Archipelago the use of betel extends west and north-west over a large part of the Pacific groups of islands, the Dutch East Indies, and from the Philippines it stretches to the banks of the Yang-Tse-Kiang, and from the east coast of Indochina, including all the islands of the Indian Ocean, to the

Indus. At the present day the Indus is the western boundary of the use of betel, although there is no doubt that in ancient times it extended to the Euphrates and part of Arabia. In a south-eastern direction the Arafura Sea and the Torres Strait seem to form an impenetrable barrier.

Betel is consumed in the following countries and islands: The most southern point where it is a popular custom is the island of Réunion. It is also a local habit in Madagascar. In Zanzibar all sections of the population chew it, even women. Opposite Zanzibar, on the East African coast, for instance on the Tanga coast, the Swahili and Arabs prefer betel to tobacco; so also do the inhabitants of the island of Mafia, the most southerly of the islands of the Zanzibar Archipelago, and the people of Hadramaut. In Persia and Baluchistan its use is not extensive. Beyond the Indus it is consumed in large quantities. The real betel countries are the Konkan Coast, Kanara, the Malabar territory as far as Cape Comorin, Travancore, the Laccadive and the Maldive Islands, Ceylon, the Coromandel Coast, Assam, Bengal, Hindustan, the Punjab, the Himalaya states, the Andamans and Nicobars, Malacca, Burma, the Shan States, Siam, Cambodia, Cochin China, Annam, Tonkin, the south and southeast coast of China, especially Yun-nan, Kwang-si, Kwang-Tung and Che-Kiang, also Kainan, the Sonda Islands, for instance Timor, Borneo, Java, Sumatra, Nias, Banka, Biliton, the Moluccas, the Banda Islands, Amboina, Buru, Ceram, Ternate, etc., the Philippines with the exception of the west coast of Palawan, Formosa, the Caroline Islands with the exception of Ponage, the Marianne Islands, New Guinea and the Louisiade Archipelago, the Hermit and Admiralty Islands, the Bismarck Archipelago, New Ireland (New Mecklenburg), New Britain (New Pomerania), Heath Island, the Solomon Islands, Bougainville, etc., Duke of York Island (New Lauenburg), the Shortlands and Santa Cruz Islands, the island of Tukopia and the Fiji Islands. The New Hebrides and New Caledonia do not seem to use the drug. Betel is only chewed on the Banks Islands and to a small extent on the Marquesas Islands.

The number of betel-chewers I estimate at about 200 million. But it is not consumed to the same extent in all parts. Its use, for instance, is more intensive on the coast of Eastern India than in the interior. In the central districts of Sumatra it is less frequent, partly on account of the lack of lime. In the north of China, betel is considered a great luxury because the plant cannot be found growing wild.

The passion for the drug is common to all, both men and women, to every age and class: princes, priests, workmen, and slaves consume it. All religions participate, Christians, especially coloured missionaries, Mohammedans, Buddhists, Brahmans, Fetishists, and other sects. All races are addicted to the drug, Caucasians, Mongols, Malays, Papuans, Alfurus, etc. Some tribes are more immoderate in its use than others. It is stated, for instance, that the Malays and Burmese are more addicted to it than the Bengalese. Among the Dorese generally only the chiefs consume betel. It is said that they acquired this habit from the Tidorese. In all cases the abuse starts in infancy and ceases with death. In Burma there is a proverb illustrating the premature use of the drug, which says that no one can speak Burmese properly until he can chew betel. It is chewed at all times, at work and rest, sitting or standing, at home and on a visit. The craving of these people for the drug may be judged from the fact that love alone is capable of making a person cease chewing for a short time. Tagalese girls regard it a sign of the sincerity and violence of their lover's passion if he removes the betel from his mouth. It is said that the betel nut is even retained during sleep. The first thing the inhabitant of New Britain seizes on awaking is areca nut and betel pepper, and he continues to chew it until far into the night. The savage of south-east New Guinea values this delight as much as sleep and dancing.

Many Europeans have become addicted to the drug.

History and Mode of Chewing Betel

So widespread a custom can be explained only by the fact that it must have had a long history. Only a continual progress of the use of betel for hundreds of years can have resulted in so vast a distribution and the penetration of the habit into all social classes as is described on the preceding pages. Indeed its use has been traced back for more than two thousand years. About 340 B.C. Theophrastus described the areca palm, whose nuts are a component of the betel morsel. This palm is also mentioned in Sanscrit under the name of *guvàka*, and is referred to in Chinese texts about 150 B.C. as *pinlang*, a Malayan name which it still bears at the present day. The betel leaf, the second essential component of the betel morsel, is already described in the most ancient historic documents of Ceylon, in the Mahávamsa, which is written in the Pali language. It is there stated that in the year 504 B.C. a princess made a present of betel to her lover. During the combat between Duthagámini and the Malabars in the year 161 B.C., his enemies remarked on his lips that blood-red colour which is caused by the chewing of betel and spread the rumor that he had been wounded.

Reports dating from the first centuries of our era also enable us to conclude that betel was extensively used in India. The Arabs and Persians who reached Hindustan in the eighth and ninth centuries found this habit deeply rooted and made it known in their own countries. The use of betel in Persia, however, is much older. The Persian historian Ferishta writes that there were 30,000 shops for the sale of betel alone, in the capital town Kanyakubia during the reign of Khosru Parviz (i.e. Chosroes II, A.D. 600). Masudi, who travelled through India in 916, describes the chewing of betel as a national custom which even those who voluntarily ascend the funeral pyre practised as a final comfort. Those who do not use betel, moreover, were socially isolated. He states that the areca nut was highly valued by the inhabitants of Mecca, Yemen, and the Hejaz, who substituted it for mastix. The famous travellers of the Middle Ages, Marco Polo for instance, who in the thirteenth century explored Central Asia, China, India, and Persia, or Ibn Batuta who travelled over the whole Mohammedan world in the fourteenth century, describe the growth of betel, how it climbs like a vine on supports of the palm-trunks. They describe how betel is used, together with the areca nut and lime, and the effects which follow. Later centuries have abundantly enriched and improved this first knowledge of the drug.

The typical betel morsel is composed of a piece of areca nut, the fruit of the palm tree *areca catechu*, in any state of maturity, a betel leaf, the leaf of *piper (chavica) betle*, and a certain amount of burnt lime. In some parts tobacco, gambir, or catechu are added, of which the last two contain tannin. In various countries differences may be ascertained in the manner in which the ingredients are introduced, their order, etc. The morsel is then eagerly pushed from one side of the mouth to the other, masticated, chewed, and pressed against or between the teeth in order to remove the juice, so that the substance frequently protrudes from between the lips.

The first apparent effect of this process of mastication is an abundant salivation. Some chewers spit out this first saliva and others swallow

it, together with the subsequent excessive secretion of saliva and betel juice. In this way they chew and chew their hardest, and in the
case of a hard nut, with a large expenditure of energy, until only a few
ligneous fibers similar to tow remain, which are ejected, the red masses
of juice being swallowed. Nevertheless, remnants of the nut can frequently be observed between the teeth.

The morsels are not always prepared extempore. On the Indian
continent and in the Indian islands ready prepared morsels are kept at
home or in the so-called betel bag. Small shops also display morsels of
this kind for sale. In Manila the female members of the family prepare
these quids (buyo). In every living-room there is a small box containing the implements and ingredients necessary for this purpose. These
buyo are chewed for approximately half an hour. In Siam, women and
children are engaged with the removal of the thin outer bark of the
fresh areca nut. Wives do this for their husbands, sisters for their broth-
ers, and girls for their lovers. If the nut is very dry and fresh ones are
not available, the Siamese prepare the betel quids as follows: They
crush the nut in a vessel similar to a mortar, which is open on both
sides. The lower opening tapers off, is narrower than the top, and is
closed with a wooden stopper. The powder of the nut is triturated
with the lime and the leaf, and pressed out of the narrow bottom of
the vessel, from which the stopper is removed, in the form of a quid.
The areca nut, betel leaf, and lime are also crushed, on the coast of
New Guinea.

The betel leaf is consumed only in a fresh state, for old ones are
without any action whatever. Light yellow leaves are preferred. Frequent moistening of the leaves keeps them fresh for a longer period.
The betel leaves presented to visitors at the courts of Indian princes
are gilded.

The quantity of the ingredients consumed daily naturally differs
with the individual. The areca nut constitutes about three-quarters of
the weight of the whole morsel, the rest being made up by the betel
leaf and the lime. In Java one of the larger betel leaves or one and a
half of the smaller leaves is used for one quid. Approximately 0.5 gr. of
lime are added. In Siam the highest quantity consumed in one day is
said to amount to fifty portions (k'āms) for an adult, equal to $12^{1}/_{2}$
nuts, and the lowest daily consumption amounts to approximately one-
fourth of this quantity. Linschoten states that men and women con-

sume 36 and more betel leaves a day. According to another report the daily average consumption in China is 24 leaves.

Of the lime, which generally is carefully kept in closed vessels, a piece the size of a pea or about 0.6 gr. is used. Sometimes more is added, up to a quarter of the weight of the morsel.

Effect of Betel-Chewing

Persons not accustomed to the chewing of betel experience a disagreeable, acrid, and burning taste, and a feeling of constriction in the throat after a very short period of mastication. Slight sores on the tongue and the throat also occur. As more betel is chewed, this at first almost intolerable sensation diminishes. Finally hardly anything of the kind is felt, and the sensations experienced are even agreeable. Bishop Heber himself declared that he quite understood why the habitués of betel liked its consumption. The perception of taste is not infrequently reduced for a short time, probably on account of the essential oil contained in the leaves, or perhaps the action of the lime. But even if it is possible for Europeans to become accustomed to the taste of betel, there is one circumstance which frequently prevents them from becoming addicted to the drug, and that is the excessive amount of saliva formed, which, especially at the beginning, obliges them to spit very frequently. This is all the more repugnant to Europeans because the saliva is yellowish-brown, brownish-red, or blood-red, according to the amount of lime used. This excessive salivation according to my own experiments has its origin in an irritation of the mouth by the ingredients of the areca nut. The colouration of the saliva is also due to the colouring matter of the nut which assumes the hues described under the influence of the alkaline lime. The usual threefold mixture, areca nut, betel leaf, and lime, furnishes a red-brown saliva, the fourfold, areca nut, betel leaf, gambir and catechu, and lime a saliva of more blood-red colour. The differences, however, are not great.

After the first effects of the excitation of the salivary glands and the irritation of the mucous membranes of the mouth have passed off, a pleasant odour remains in the mouth. This has always been considered one of the charms of betel-chewing. The betel leaf alone does not give rise to this smell. The odour which it produces is aromatic, but not in the least agreeable. It is the areca nut alone to which this effect is due. My experiments proved that an odoriferous substance is formed by the action of the lime on the nut, which in minute quantities has an extremely agreeable flavour. The latter is very lasting if, for instance, a few drops of the concentrated solution in ether are brought in contact with the hands or clothes. In the mouth the same effect can be observed, but to a far less degree. I can well imagine that betel is chewed on account of this odour and agreeable taste. This opinion should not be objected to on the ground that many old and inveterate betel-chewers in Siam exhale an extremely unpleasant breath which, on account of its peculiarity, is called "betel smell." It is stated to be so intense that the windward side is preferred when speaking with such people. This pungent smell is caused by the decomposition of small pieces of the morsel stuck between the teeth if the latter are not cleaned. Nevertheless, such persons still experience the agreeable smell and taste developed by the betel quid, and continue to chew betel in spite of the putrefaction in their mouths, or perhaps even, at a later stage, on account of it. Moreover, Jagor never noticed a bad smell from the breath of betel-chewers, and stated that it would be desirable for this custom to exist in Europe also, where foul breath is a frequent evil, especially in older persons. In inveterate betel-chewers who do not keep themselves very clean, a crust, mainly consisting of calcium carbonate, is formed in the course of time on the teeth and gums. In the Admiralty Islands the formation of this "tooth-stone" is regarded as an attribute of the dignity of chief, for only the very rich are in a position to indulge so freely in chewing as to produce such quantities of "tooth-stone." When the mouth is closed these dental excrescense protrude from between the lips like the point of a black tongue. According to Vogel the vanity of these tribes enables them to tolerate this ornament, though the teeth become loose and of hardly any use for the mastication of solid food.

The chewing of betel, however, which is practised with such intensity by so many people, must have other results besides perfuming the breath. This is indeed the case, for it produces effects on the brain. The nature and intensity of this action seem to depend upon the species and degree of maturity of the nut and also on the greater or lesser habituation to betel. As a rule betel can be considered from this point of view as a mild excitant with narcotic and stimulating properties. The betel-chewer experiences a feeling of well-being. He is in a good humour and gay, he is very little if at all bored, and is, according to the statements of Burmese monks, inspired to self-reflection and to work if he has the disposition thereto. But all this is not more pronounced than the effects of tobacco taken in any of its various forms. The famous explorer Kaempfer stated that according to his personal experiences with betel it has a soothing effect and gives rise to an excellent humour on account of its slightly inebriating action on the brain. The assumption that a more powerful narcotic action is present is not correct. I consider the statement that the betel-chewing of the Singhalese has the same effects as opium very exaggerated. On the other hand, those who chew betel for the first time in the countries of its production seem to experience very characteristic cerebral effects. The degree of maturity of the substances used is probably a decisive factor in these cases. According to the statements of those who themselves experienced the effects of the drug, its results are similar to those of tobacco. Uneasiness, a stifling sensation, especially faintness, slight excitation, a kind of inebriety, outbreak of sweat, and occasionally torpor are the symptoms liable to occur. They are not of long duration, and after habituation is established they are said not to appear again.

The feeling of thirst and hunger is said to be appeased and the sexual impulses augmented by the chewing of betel. This last, however, is not correct.

It is of the utmost importance to know whether the permanent use of mixtures containing betel has consequences injurious to the organism similar to those produced by the majority of other narcotics. I myself believe that the harmlessness of betel may be confirmed, even in cases of excessive use. From a toxicological point of view the objections which can be made to its use are less serious than, for instance, those against alcohol and tobacco. Taken as a whole, the ill consequences of betel are relatively so trifling that we might wish that the devotees of other substances of the same kind experienced as little inconvenience. Naturally all such addictions have one thing in common; after the habit has been established to the habitués are slaves to their passion. Habit leads to necessity and necessity to constraint. Every constraint reduces individual liberty, especially if it is exercised on organic life, for it soon leads to the imperative craving of certain cellular groups for a repetition of the agreeable excitation. From this point of view the consumption of betel must indeed be regarded as an evil. It must also be taken into consideration that if chewers of betel abstain from its use for some reason or other, withdrawal symptoms

set in which are different in nature and intensity from those called
forth by the deprivation of other narcotics. General fatigue, exhaustion, and weakness occur because the digestive organs are not stimulated by the drug. An unpleasant taste occurs in the mouth and the
breath is foul. Other organic disorders due to weakness are liable to
show themselves.

These advantages lose in importance if they are compared with
the agreeable sensations due to betel and the resistance against injurious climatic influences which this substance gives to its users. Thanks
to an inexplicable instinct the natives of the Far East discovered the
action of this tonic agent as a means of protection against the ill effects of their food. With the exception of bread-fruit and some species
of leguminous plants, their food contains hardly any nitrogen. An
excess of acid decomposition products of this over-uniform food is
very liable to formation in the stomach. The alkaline juice of the
betel morsel neutralizes this acidity and acts as an astringent, harden-
ing the mucous membranes of the stomach. We can adhere without
question to the opinion that no medical prescription is apt to attain
the desired result better than betel. All who have investigated the
conditions of life in tropical countries have come to the conclusion
that the moderate chewing of betel only promotes health, especially
when considered in relation to the primitive and miserable food of
the Indians and the frequently terrible climatic conditions. The fact
that most Europeans abstain from betel without injury to their health
proves nothing, for their food is quite different and they take sufficient alcoholic excitants. Nevertheless, many of them suffer from various disorders of the digestive organs, general weakness, prostration,
and dysentery, which would probably not occur if betel were used.

To which element of the betel morsel is the exciting action on
the nervous system? The answer to this question is easily given. It is
for the main part the areca nut which contains a substance which is
active in this direction, the oily, volatile arecoline.

By experimentation on animals it has been ascertained that this
substance produces states of excitation of the central nervous system,
for instance an increase of the excitability of the reflexes and eventually convulsions succeeded by paralysis. The mucous membranes are
also irritated (salivation, liquid stools). Respiration is more frequent
and the work of the heart diminished. The action on the nervous

system is not always the same, and many differences depending on individual or general disposition can be ascertained. Dogs, for instance, after ingestion of areca nut exhibit a state of extreme excitation; frogs, on the other hand, symptoms of depression. The quality of the nut also seems to be of importance. In man it has been observed that after the consumption of a certain species of nuts, especially when not quite ripe, a state of vertigo appears which is similar to that experienced under the influence of wine. The condition produced by nuts of this kind has in Siam its own name, *San Makh.*[2] I have, however, already stated that old nuts frequently give rise to cerebral symptoms. Without a doubt this modification in the action is due to the proportion of arecoline content in the nut.

The essential oil in the betel leaf produces, according to my experiments on animals, a primary excitation followed by a kind of inebriety. It plays a secondary part in the action of the betel morsel on the nerves. We must also take into consideration that the more alkaline the lime, the more will the arecoline alkaloid be liberated from the areca nut, i.e. in proportion to the calcium hydrate content of the lime employed.

KAT

My friend G. Schweinfurth wrote to me as follows: "When during my travels in Yemen I saw the high, many-storied houses of the mountain villages late at night brilliantly illuminated, and their windows shining in the darkness, I enquired what the inhabitants did at that time of the night. I was told that 'friends and acquaintances meet and sit for hours round the brazier drinking their coffee prepared from the husks[3] and chew their indispensable kat, which keeps them awake and promotes friendly intercourse.'"

The kat-eater is happy when he hears everyone talk in turn and tries to contribute to this social entertainment. In this way the hours pass in a rapid and agreeable manner. Kat produces joyous excitation and gaiety. Desire for sleep is banished, energy is revived during the hot hours of the day, and the feeling of hunger on long marches is dispersed. Messengers and warriors use kat because it makes the ingestion of food unnecessary for several days.

The above-described effects, which remind one of those of caffeine plants, are due to the mastication of the young buds and the fresh leaves of *catha edulis* (*celastrus edulis*), a large shrub which can be grown to the size of a tree. It is only cultivated for consumption in the cool valleys situated at a height of 900 to 1,200 metres in north-east Africa and south-west Arabia and Abyssinia. It is cultivated to a great extent in Harar, Tigre, Shoa, Kafa, Yemen, etc. The northern limit of occurrence of kat is approximately 18° north latitude. It may be found in a wild state up to about 30° south latitude in Natal and Pondoland. The spread of Islam in the Galla countries has led to an increase of the consumption of kat, but not to its cultivation.

Kat (*cātō*, khat among the Amhara, *ćat* or *jimma* among the Oromó) was employed in Yemen even before coffee. The mode of application has not changed. The fresh green points of the leaves, and the shoots of the leaves and stems are eaten, and it is only in Arabia that an infusion of the plant is prepared. The passion for the drug is so great that even material sacrifices are made in order to indulge in it. There are epicures in Hodeida, Mocha, and Aden who spend two dollars a day on kat. An explorer reported that the Sheikh Hassan of Yemen consumed more than 100 francs worth of kat per day because he was accustomed to have many distinguished visitors. There is a special kat market in Aden, where many people from Yemen live as workmen, merchants, etc. The plant does not grown on the plain, and express messengers have to bring it during the night in bundles from the mountains to the market. Forty branches are tied together in a bundle and inserted into a sheath which is carefully prepared from banana-leaves or palm-leaves in order to keep the material fresh during the long horse ride to market. In some places, for instance in Harar, the consumption of kat is intimately connected with the observance of prayers. The Harari, the Mohammedan Oromó, the Kafficho, the Galla, etc., are also addicted to kat. The plant is also consumed in Eyssaland and is imported from Harar and Arabia. The chewing of kat is quite unknown in Hedjaz and in Jeddah.

The active element of kat is stated to be an alkaloid which occurs in quantities varying from 0.07 per cent to 0.12 per cent in the best plants. Certain analogies with several medicinal plants have led me to the conclusion that the essential oil or resin, similar to cinnamic esters, which is also contained in the plant takes part in the peculiar exciting action.

Kat, like all other powerful substances when excessively abused, inevitably gives rise to more or less serious consequences. Those organic functions which are incessantly subjected to the influence of the drug finally flag or are diverted into another channel of activity. And kat is indeed excessively employed by high and low. The kat-eater is seized with a restlessness which robs him of sleep. The excited cerebral hemispheres do not return to their normal state of repose, and in consequence the functions of the peripheral organs, especially those of the heart, suffer to such a degree that serious cardiac affections have been ascertained in a great number of kat-eaters. The disorders of the nervous system in many cases also give rise to troubles of general metabolism partly due to the chronic loss of appetite from the consumption of kat.

Schweinfurth told me that in no part of the Mohammedan East had he seen so many bachelors as in Yemen. In other countries of Islam this state is regarded as shameful. In Yemen it was openly stated that inveterate eaters of kat were indifferent to sexual excitation and desire, and did not marry at all, or for economic reasons waited until they had saved enough money. The loss of libido sexualis has been also observed in other inhabitants of these countries.

Mohammedan casuists have frequently discussed the question whether the consumption of kat is contrary to the law of the Koran which prohibits the use of wine and everything that inebriates. Even had they come to the conclusion that kat belongs to those substances, no kat-eater would have renounced his passion.

The use of kat has become a permanent custom. Originating in Abyssinia, where it was mentioned for the first time in the year 1332, the plant penetrated into Yemen and other parts. There is no doubt that kat was consumed a long time before the date indicated, and will continue to be used in the future, for excitants of the brain defy the lapse of time.

CAFFEINE PLANTS

In the case of all substances with agreeable effects on the brain we are presented with the same problem: In what mysterious way or with the aid of what instinct has man been able to select from the immense vegetable world the plant most suitable and desirable for his purposes? Is it pure chance which led him to the discovery of a substance which he did not look for but which experience alone taught him to consider very precious? We may assume that in prehistoric times someone accidentally swallowed the milky juice of the poppy, fell asleep, and subsequently passed on the knowledge of the action of opium, or that an inhabitant of Kamchatka ate an agaric in order to vary the monotony of his food, experienced hallucinations and visions, and induced others to use it also, or that a North American Indian consumed an *anhalonium lewinii* out of curiosity. In every one of these cases we have a single vegetable product with a chemical structure and action appertaining only to this one plant, and possessed by no other natural product.

When, however, following this line of research and deliberation, we arrive at plants which owe their exciting effects on the brain to their content of caffeine or similar purine derivatives, all these suppositions and assumptions become void and meaningless. For we are confronted by the fact that man has discovered morphologically quite different plants in three of the largest continents of the world, America, Africa, and Asia, which all combine the sole and all-important feature, a content of caffeine. These plants not only play a considerable part in the organic life of the individual, but have reached a stage of capital importance for whole races and for all the world, owing to the important production and exchange of goods to which they give rise. By what long and mysterious path has man all over the world reached the same final result? How did it happen that the Arab of Yemen or of Arabia Felix not only discovered the coffee bean, but also its exciting properties, and learnt and taught others how to prepare it? By what means did the inhabitants of the Sudan gain their knowledge of the effects of the kola nut, which also contains caffeine? How did it come about that the inhabitants of the Far East highly valued the tea plant and learnt its proper preparation in order to obtain a caffeine beverage? How did the South Americans of Brazil and Paraguay, out of the thousands of equatorial and subequatorial plants, recognize a species of ilex as the vegetable product suited to supply a beverage which owes its cerebral effects to its caffeine content? And why does the Indian of the Amazon employ *paullinia sorbilis* on account of the caffeine contained therein?

The inconceivable has proved true: though man did not consciously search for the substance, and though experimental investigation was out of the question, he discovered the best possible plant, both in the Arabian Peninsula and in the wild and unexplored Matto Grosso, up to the Parana. He found it in the fever-stricken virgin forests of the Amazon and in the basin of the great Niger. We shall easily understand that Orientals especially see some mystery in this unconscious discovery, and frequently give it a mythical origin. Fables of this kind at least cast over the insoluble problem the charm of poetic illusion, whereas prosaic reality and science must respond with a brutal "We do not know" to the important question of the origin of the mysterious coincidences revealed by the use of substances containing caffeine throughout the whole world.

We know in fact that man has attached himself tenaciously to the caffeine plants and their derivatives and daily satisfies the desire they have inspired in him. And this for good reasons. An abyss separates the properties and action of these plants from those of the other substances described in this work. Consciousness is not obscured by a veil of dimness or darkness, the individual is not degraded by the destruction of his free will to animal instincts, and the soul and mental powers are not excited to the inward perception of phantasms. The caffeine plants exercise an exciting action on the brain without giving rise to any mentally or physically painful impressions. All these facts assign a particular place to these substances.

COFFEE

History of its Use

The conquest of the world by coffee must have taken place with a prodigious rapidity if what an Arabic manuscript in the National Library in Paris records be true. The Sheikh Abd-al-Kader ben Mohamed states in the sixteenth century that coffee was not in general use in Yemen as a popular beverage before the middle of the fifteenth century. If this be so, four and a half centuries have sufficed to extend its use over the whole world!

According to Abd-al-Kader ben Mohamed there lived in Aden a Mufti, Jemal-ed-din Dhabhani, who on a journey to the west coast of the Red Sea became acquainted with the use of coffee and its medicinal application. He made it known in his home country, and pilgrims brought it to Mecca and the rest of Arabia. This statement may be believed without altering our view that coffee had been known for a long time to the Arabs or the Persians as a substance endowed with marvellous properties, and was presented by the Archangel Gabriel to Mohammed when he was sick. It was even known to ease the brain and to prevent sleep. The discovery of these effects very early became the subject of many legends.

According to the Maronite Faustus Nairo, the prior of a Mohammedan convent was told by his shepherds that goats who had eaten the beans of the coffee plant remained awake and jumped and gambolled about at night. This gave him the idea of preparing a beverage for himself and his dervishes in order to keep awake during the long night prayers in the Mosque. The beverage was called *kahweh*, i.e. that which stimulates or suppresses the appetite for food. In this way it was attempted, not for the first time, to explain the initial discovery of the effects by an accidental occurrence at some remote period in Arabia.

Did the great Arab physician Avicenna in the year 1000 refer to coffee as *bunc* or *bunco*? Did Rhazes mention it 100 years earlier? By the Amhara in Abyssinia at the present day an infusion of coffee is called *buno* or *bun*, and the Oromó call it *safira buno*. The fact that the Crusaders did not mention the use of coffee need not be taken into consideration. They had other things to do, such as massacring Jews, Greeks and Turks, and bathing in blood after the fall of Jerusalem. Besides, they did not penetrate into what if only for this reason is well called "Arabia Felix." They did not even reach Abyssinia, where coffee was employed at a very early date. The Arabs frequently pointed out that they had obtained coffee from that country. I believe that the use of such substances remains a local custom for some time before it spreads. This must have been especially the case in ancient times when a continuous connection between countries difficult of access existed hardly or not at all. In the year 1511 the Egyptian Sultan appointed a new governor of Mecca. The latter did not know of coffee, and was highly displeased when one day he saw some dervishes sitting in a corner of the mosque drinking it in order to be able to carry out the ascetic exercises of the night without falling asleep. He drove them away and called a meeting of theologians, jurists, and notables of the town in order to discuss whether coffee is an inebriant. They disputed for a long time. One of those present made the whole assembly burst out laughing by stating that coffee was similar in its action to wine. He proved by this statement that he had drunk wine against the law of the Koran, and was condemned to a certain number of strokes on the soles of his feet as prescribed for this infringement of the law. As the assembly could not come to a decision they had recourse to two physicians, who stated that coffee was injurious and was apt to give rise to actions which were improper for a Mohammedan. The meeting condemned it, prohibited its sale, and burnt all they could find. Those convicted of having drunk coffee were led through the town mounted on a donkey. This prohibition, however, was soon abolished, for the Sultan of Cairo was an avid coffee-drinker and his wise counsellors declared it admissible and harmless. Twenty years later, after the use of coffee had become very popular in Cairo, a new campaign was inaugurated against it, and it was declared that a coffee-drinker could not be a good Mohammedan. The excitement which these sermons caused gave rise to the devastation of coffee-shops, etc. The religious leaders repeatedly tried in later times to raise an agitation against coffee. But all opposition finally succumbed, and a Turkish law even decided that the refusal of a husband to give his wife coffee is a legal ground for divorce. Coffee had been victorious. Its road free from obstacles, it was enabled to march forward and conquer the countries of the world, which indeed it did.

The physician Rauwolf[4] of Augsburg on his journeys in Asia Minor, Syria, and Persia in the years 1573 to 1578 found that coffee was used there by the entire population as if it were an ancient custom. Indeed the first coffee-house in Constantinople had been established in the reign of Suleiman in 1551. Rauwolf states:

> Among other things they possess a beverage which they value highly, called chaube. It is as black as ink, and very useful in various diseases, especially those of the stomach. They usually take it in the morning in public without fear of being seen. They drink it from small earthen or porcelain cups, as hot as they can bear it. They frequently lift these vessels to their lips and take small sips, and then pass them round in the order in which they are sitting. They prepare the beverage from water and a fruit which the natives call

bunnu. This somewhat resembles the laurel berry in size and colour. This beverage is very much in use, and for this reason a large number of merchants may be seen in the bazaars selling the fruits or the beverage.

The coffee beverage had already by this time vanquished Asia Minor and Egypt and supplanted other products. The Turkish poet Belighi[5]expresses this as follows.

> In Damascus, Aleppo and in the residence of Cairo
> It has gone round with a great Hallo!
> The coffee-bean, the scent of ambrosia!
> Then it entered the seraglio and the air of the Bosphorus,
> Seducing Doctors, Cadis and the Koran
> To sects and martyrdom!—and now
> It has triumphed! It supplanted
> In this happy hour, in the Moslem empire,
> Wine which until then was consumed!

Europe was soon numbered among the patrons of coffee.

Coffee reached Paris in 1643, and in 1690 there were already 250 coffee-houses. In the reign of Louis XV 600 had been established, and in 1782 there were 1,800. In 1702, there was in that city a luxuriously installed café with tapestries, large mirrors on the walls, crystal chandeliers, and marble tables where coffee as well as tea and chocolate were served. This luxury contributed much to the extension of the use of coffee to all classes of society. Nevertheless, it was opposed on many hands. In her famous letters to her daughter, Madame de Grignan, Madame de Sevigné frequently points out the varying opinions of coffee held by herself and others on account of the different reports of medical men, etc., on the subject. And what was not said about its effects! In 1697 it was recommended in a Paris medical dissertation. In 1715 it was proved in the same city that it shortens life. In 1716 its property of facilitating intellectual work was praised, and in 1718 the fact that it does not produce apoplexy. At a later date it was stated to cause inflammation of the liver and spleen and renal colic, to have ruined the stomach of the minister Colbert, etc. It is remarkable that a physician at that period had already noticed the action of coffee on the circulation of the blood and the evil effects it is liable to produce when abused at night in order to keep awake for work. At the beginning of the eighteenth century coffee had penetrated into the life of many peoples and cities, though sometimes not without difficulty. The opposition to coffee commenced in the year 1511, but only here and there was it of long duration, and never so in Germany where several small potentates, not content with prohibiting coffee, even offered a reward to the informer. One of these, the Prince of Waldeck by the grace of God, paid ten thalers to anyone who should denounce a coffee-drinker. Even laundrywomen and ironers were rewarded if they laid information against their employers from whom they had obtained coffee. Several punishments were introduced against sellers of coffee in the small towns and in the country. Men of note were allowed to buy coffee in the capital cities. In 1777 the Prince-Bishop Wilhelm of Paderborn declared that the drinking of coffee was a privilege of the aristocracy, the clergy, and the high officials. It was strictly prohibited to the middle classes and the peasants. Drinkers of coffee in Germany were even threatened with caning. As the use of coffee increased in Prussia King Frederick II imposed a high tax on it. The people must again become accustomed to drinking beer on which "His Royal Majesty himself" had, according to the edict, been brought up. In his opinion this was far healthier than coffee. In a comedy by Kotzebue, a husband praises the economy of his young wife in the following words: "Have I not given up coffee? Have I not sighed in the morning when drinking my beer, because, as Hufeland says, our forefathers derived much benefit from it?"

However, substances which act on the brain mock at all obstacles which oppose their extension. Their attraction grows slowly, silently, but surely. Finally, even the authors of legal restrictions themselves become an easy prey to the fascination of these excitants. Coffee has fulfilled its destiny, and it may be that countless souls who enjoyed its influence on this earth yearn for it in the world to come.

Cultivation and Use

The cultivation of coffee rapidly spread over tropical and subtropical countries. In the middle of the eighteenth century the Franciscan friar Villaso planted some coffee-plants in the garden of the San Antonio convent in Rio de Janeiro, and from there Jesuits and Capuchins brought it to the missions of São Paolo. At the beginning of this century the export from Brazilian ports alone amounted to 12 to 14 millions sacks of coffee, containing 60 kilos per sack. The State of São Paolo, together with Minas Gerães, produces more than double the quantity raised in the other coffee-growing countries—Africa, India, the Dutch East Indies, Central America, Venezuela, and the Antilles. The consumption of coffee varies in different countries and periods. Table 8 shows the amount of coffee consumed by a number of countries in 1912.

TABLE 8. AMOUNT OF COFFEE CONSUMED IN 1912

COUNTRY	AMOUNT
North America	more than 7 million sacks (of 60 kg.)
Germany	more than 3 million sacks (of 60 kg.)
France	more than $1^3/_4$ million sacks (of 60 kg.)
Austria-Hungary	more than 1 million sacks (of 60 kg.)
Holland	5 kg. per head annually

Taxes on coffee and severe economic conditions have greatly re- duced the import and consumption of the beverage in Germany. How- ever, the curve is rising again, although the use of tea and cocoa con- tinues to increase annually. The very instructive Table 9 not only il- lustrates the increase and decrease of the use of coffee but also gives information as to the countries of origin.

The absolute coercion which is imposed on the Americans of the United States by the Prohibition Act with respect to alcohol has nec- essarily had the result of greatly increasing the use of other excitants and also narcotics. The enormous abuse of the latter seems to be to- tally ignored by the abstainers in America. Morphinists and cocainists are continually growing in numbers. The consumption of coffee has also developed in an undreamt-of manner. In 1919 421 million kilos were consumed and in 1920 as many as 616 million kilos. The con- sumption therefore increased from 4 to 9 kilos per head per year, and is approaching the threshold of abuse.

Coffee is employed over the whole world. A few bodies prohibit its use, for instance the Senüssi, an important sect in the Lybian desert and the Oasis of Ammon, founded in the eighteenth century by Sidi Mohammed ben ali es-Senüssi. They also refrain from smoking. Tea is allowed them, and they sweeten it with cane-sugar, because crystal- lized sugar is unclean, having been refined with the bones of animals (animal charcoal) killed by unbelievers.[6] The nomadic tribes of Syria, however, drink freshly roasted coffee which they import from Yemen. They do not add sugar, but spice it with cardamon.

Effects of Coffee

> O coffee, thou dost disperse cares and sorrows, thou art the drink of
> the friends of God, thou givest health to those who labour to obtain
> wisdom. Only the reasonable man, he who drinks coffee, knows the
> truth. Coffee is our gold; where it is offered us we enjoy the com-
> pany of the best people. God grant that the obstinate despisers of
> the beverage may never taste its pleasures.

This inspired hymn of coffee was written for posterity by an enthusiastic lover of the beverage, the Sheikh Abd al-Kader, 400 years ago.
Another poet sings of coffee as the destroyer of care and sorrow, as the
water with which solicitude is washed away, the fire which consumes
it.[7] These exaggerated glorifications from the Orient and the more
cautious praise of poets of Western countries at a later period are opposed by bitter criticisms of coffee, just as one-sided as the commen-
dations. At the end of the seventeenth century, for instance, the famous naturalist Redi[8] concludes a dithyramb in praise of Tuscan wine
by a sharp censure of the coffee-drinker. He would rather drink poison
than a glass of the bitter and injurious coffee, which was invented by
the Belides and given to Proserpine by the Furies, and which now,
black as night in colour, has become the favourite beverage of the
injudicious Arabs and Janizzaries:

> *Beverei prima il veleno,*
> *Che un bicchier, che fosse pieno*
> *Dell' amaro, e reo Caffe:*
> *Colà tra gli Arabi,*
> *E tra i Gianizzeri,*
> *Liquor sì ostico.*
> *Sì nero, e torbido.*
> *Gli schiavi ingollino.*
> *Giu nel Tartaro,*
> *Giu nell' Erebo,*
> *L' empie Belidi l'inventarono,*
> *E Tesifone, e l'altre Furie*
> *A Proserpina il ministrarono;*
> *E se in Asia il Musulmanno*
> *Se lo cionca a precipizio,*
> *Mostra aver poco giudizic.*

TABLE 9. IMPORT OF RAW COFFEE INTO GERMANY

AMOUNT IN DOUBLE-CENTNERS OF 100 KG.

COUNTRY OF ORIGIN	1911	1912	1913	1920	1921	1922	1923	1924	1925
British East Africa	525	589	217	906	4,548	906	1,000	1,402	1,082
German East Africa	5,419	3,443	3,996	43	793	174	80	706	519
Liberia	500	395	311	202	285	61	211	308	179
Portuguese West Africa	6,257	3,567	1,709	5	1,586	1,123	455	193	1,066
Arabia	—	—	—	—	—	146	537	1,206	1,844
British India	22,287	22,010	28,989	3,945	7,595	650	2,870	7,554	13,718
Dutch East Indies	41,306	51,313	58,520	64,807	67,439	25,855	5,312	26,331	36,229
Brazil	1,413,933	1,272,993	1,159,494	297,907	793,909	268,406	289,479	266,189	389,946
Colombia	21,759	78,753	27,928	2,435	7,572	3,022	2,056	7,162	25,724
Costa Rica	26,704	22,668	29,633	2,807	9,740	1,395	2,935	24,657	43,934
Cuba	—	—	—	—	—	162	11	272	287
Guatemala	170,189	183,613	215,361	12,946	99,034	43,465	46,746	125,925	192,368
Honduras	1,500	1,812	1,771	229	896	154	268	511	641
Mexico	30,759	28,609	41,427	5,162	6,553	3,962	6,414	19,044	56,861
Nicaragua	7,452	6,309	7,298	617	2,345	100	323	2,517	4,991
Haiti	3,698	4,152	2,257	518	500	36	58	680	2,100
Salvador	25,509	20,669	30,101	976	6,147	9,222	11,804	32,228	62,129
Venezuela	35,147	49,336	56,944	6,528	21,715	7,808	15,265	27,902	52,232
U.S.A.	4,378	4,269	3,317	2,144	2,367	234	991	6,321	15,391
TOTAL	1,831,902	1,708,671	1,682,504	405,724	1,037,367	367,963	387,309	553,271	904,430

He repudiated these verses, however, towards the end of his life, and confessed to having become a coffee-drinker, who in the morning, instead of eating, drank one or two cups of the beneficial beverage "che mi toglie la sete, mi conforta lo stomaco, e mi fa altri beni."

The same conversion overtook others, among them Frederick II. What, then, is the truth?

Certainly not the statements sometimes made by persons ignorant of toxicology:[9] "The brotherhood of tea- and coffee-drinkers is subjected to the tyranny of a passion which is just as blameworthy as that of the drinkers of wine and spirits." From a scientific and practical point of view nothing is more erroneous than this, for it shows a false conception of the fundamental differences in the action of the two groups of substances. But who is there nowadays who does not consider himself in a position to give an opinion on purely toxicological problems! The habitual drinking of infusions of caffeine plants cannot be called blameworthy, for it does not in any way disturb the personality of the individual. Coffee exercises a stimulating action on the brain which results in an increased activity, whereas spirits habitually taken chemically modify the brain, as I have already pointed out. Alcohol in excess, being a morbific factor for the cerebral chemistry, imposes on the organism among other things the supplementary duty of repairing the trouble as long as it is capable of doing so. Caffeine beverages do not cause the drinker to deteriorate either physically or mentally. Even in cases where evident abuse of the beverage has taken place, the functional disorders are with a few exceptions soon adjusted.

I pointed out long ago the symptoms apt to appear after abuse of this kind.[10] These are an excessive state of brain-excitation which becomes manifest by a remarkable loquacity sometimes accompanied by accelerated association of ideas. This state occurs not infrequently at coffee-parties where gossip runs apace among the females. It may also be observed in coffee-house politicians who drink cup after cup of black coffee and by this abuse are inspired to profound wisdom on all earthly events.

Other symptoms are not lacking in those countries where alcohol is restricted and cafés have been established as a kind of compensation. Such consequences, as I have stated earlier, may, of course, take on an unpleasant character. The persons, for instance, who are regular customers of these establishments and drink coffee in excessive quantities also involuntarily consume any substances with which the beverage has been adulterated. These latter probably play a part in the occasional appearance of functional disorders. But it is not necessary to draw attention to the fact that the daily consumption of very large amounts of concentrated infusions even of pure coffee over a long period must occasionally give rise to more or less evil consequences. These are not only due to the aromatic substances formed during the roasting process, such as caffeol, pyridin, furfurol, furfuraldehyde, mono- and trimethylamin, etc., but also to caffeine itself. Gastric disorders, headaches, a state of nervous excitation with insomnia or restlessness by which the heart is sometimes affected may occur. Less frequently a state of general weakness accompanied by depression or trembling of the muscles may be ascertained. I have observed as rather unusual symptoms diplopia or weakness of sight, tinnitus aurium, agina pectoris, dyspnœa, pains in the testicles, and prostatitis.

It has frequently been stated that the drinking of coffee diminishes sexual excitability and gives rise to sterility. Though this is a mere fable, it was believed in former times. Olearius says in the account of his travels that the Persians drink "the hot, black water Chawae" whose property it is "to sterilise nature and extinguish carnal desires." A Sultan was so greatly attracted by coffee that he became tired of his wife. The latter one day saw a stallion being castrated and declared that it would be better to give the animal coffee, as then it would be in the same state as her husband. The Princess Palatine Elizabeth Charlotte (Liselotte) of Orleans, the mother of the dissipated Regent Philip II, wrote to her sisters: "Coffee is not so necessary for Protestant ministers as for Catholic priests, who are not allowed to marry and must remain chaste . . . I am surprised that so many people like coffee, for it has a bitter and bad taste. I think it tastes exactly like foul breath."

Nansen has pointed out the consequences of the abuse of coffee among the inhabitants of Greenland. They drink the beverage in a very strong state, and seldom less than two cups at a time four or five times a day. This in their own opinion is why they suffer from vertigo and are unable to hold themselves straight up in their kayaks. In order to avoid this the young men take only a little coffee or none at all.

Caffeine, which is present in coffee up to 2.5 per cent, is the principal agent which gives rise to symptoms of this kind. This has been proved by the observation of patients who consumed excessive doses of medicinally applied caffeine. The condition of cerebral excitation may increase until delirium appears. If caffeine is consumed in spirits, the evil consequences of alcohol already described are augmented. It can be stated with certainty that large quantities of caffeine are exported to America for this purpose.

Professional occupation with coffee, for instance, that of a coffee-maker who prepares and serves the beverage himself, is liable to give rise to a state of chronic excitation, for instance, in the form of delirium, vertigo, trembling, and even convulsions. This was observed in a man who had been a coffee-maker for forty years. The manageress of a coffee shop had gradually become accustomed to consume 40 coffee beans a day in order to judge the relative merits of different sorts of coffee. After four years attacks of convulsion with loss of consciousness set in. Very little is known of the consequences which the consumption of coffee-beans is liable to produce. It is practised by the Galla, who roast the powdered coffee with butter and eat it or chew the beans raw. In Unyoro and Uganda the beans are consumed whole.

The personal disposition plays a very important part in the manifestation of the undesirable effects of coffee. The evil properties which many persons attribute to coffee and other substances containing caffeine are nothing else but the consequence of their own constitution, or innate or acquired idiosyncrasies which evoke in them abnormal reactions. If persons suffer from symptoms of acute stupor after smelling odoriferous plants such as violets, roses, lilies, etc., this is not the fault of the plant, but the cause must be sought in the individuals themselves. The odour of the rotting apples which Schiller kept in the drawer of his desk caused Goethe, who sat at the desk in its owner's absence, to suffer from a state of depression with loss of consciousness. In this case it was not the properties of the apples which gave rise to this phenomenon but the particular sensibility of Goethe. If strawberries, raspberries, cinnamon, oranges, crabs, or fresh pork cause cutaneous eruptions, sickness with vomiting, or attacks of asthma to appear in some persons, the foodstuffs in question cannot be considered responsible. I was the first to describe these individual states of increased sensitivity,[11] and thus gave occasion to many expositions on the same subject. A hypersensitivity to coffee, which may be the expression of a kind of cellular weakness, may occur in some person and characterizes the individual and not the coffee. When Goethe observed of himself that the heavy beer of Merseburg obscured his ideas and that coffee, especially when taken with milk after meals, gave rise in him to a peculiarly sad humour, paralysed his intestines and seemed to suspend their functions, which caused him great anxiety, then the reason for these particular phenomena must be sought in Goethe himself.

Objections cannot be raised to the use of coffee on account of the phenomena described on the preceding pages. The evil consequences which its abusive employment in the form of the bean, the pulp of the beans, or the husks, which latter are used for the preparation of an infusion (*kisher*) in Yemen and the Galla country, are exceptions which in no way justify a deprecatory opinion of the use of coffee as a stimulant. It exercises a gently stimulating influence on the brain, and in this way the propensity to sleep is diminished. Mental capacity and perhaps also the imagination are agreeably augmented. Coffee inhibits the appearance of fatigue, or at least makes it less perceptible, and in this way tends to increase the capacity for work and the general activity without exerting any violent force on the cerebral centres. In the same gentle manner the activity of the heart in healthy persons is augmented. As soon as these effects become evident a feeling of general depression and weakness may be dispersed and the working capacity of the muscles stimulated for a certain time. This state is not succeeded by a subjective feeling of subsequent fatigue. It is an open question whether the process of metabolism is modified in any direction, as some have stated. The personal experience of millions of coffee-drinkers in all parts of the world testifies to the stimulating action described. The manifestations of the latter are known, but its ultimate causes, as is the case with so many phenomena in this field, remain undiscovered.

TEA

In the year 519, Darma, the third son of the Indian king Kosyuvo, landed in China. He was an apostle of the religion which the Indian sage Sakya had founded and spread throughout the Far East. He lived constantly under the open sky, mortified his flesh, and tamed his passions. His food consisted of leaves, and he sought the most profound degree of sanctity by staying awake all night in uninterrupted meditation on the Divine Being. After many years it happened that, worn out with fatigue from his long mortifications, he was overcome by sleep. On waking he felt so full of remorse for having broken his vow that, resolving to prevent forever a repetition of this weakness, he cut off both his eyelids, the instruments of his sin, and cast them away in abhorrence. On the following day, when he came back to the place of his pious suffering, he found that a plant had miraculously sprung forth from the spot where his eyelids had fallen. It was the tea-plant. He ate the leaves, and soon experienced a feeling of joy and gladness, and was able to plunge into the contemplation of the Divine Being with renewed activity and vigour. He explained the effects of the leaves of tea and their mode of consumption to his disciples, and the fame of the plant soon spread and became generally known.

This Chinese fable seeks to explain by a miracle how man became acquainted with the stimulating properties of the tea-plant, which, like coffee, contains caffeine. In this case, as in many others of the same kind, man instinctively feels it impossible to find the origin of the first recognition of the effects of the plant, and has shrouded the events of the past in the veil of a myth. In reality tea must have been known at an extremely early age. Near Urga in Mongolia vestiges of prehistoric man several thousand years old, the bones of hitherto unknown animals, and in one of the tombs tea and cereal have been discovered.

It was not till the end of the sixteenth century that the rest of the world became acquainted with the properties of tea, although it has been extensively employed in China since the fifth century, if not earlier. It is difficult to say whether the knowledge of tea originated in China or whether it came from India, especially from Assam. Towards the end of the eighth century, in the time of the Tang dynasty, taxes on tea were first imposed. At the beginning of the ninth century it reached Japan. In the meantime, before penetrating into Europe it must have continued its triumphant march towards Tibet and Mongolia, and thence in a westerly and easterly direction. In these parts it became known as a stimulating beverage to explorers of the Far East such as Ramusio, Ludovico Almeida, etc. In 1636 tea was

drunk in Paris, and in 1646 the East India Company sent 90 gr. of it to
King Charles II of England. Some time later one kilo was sold for £3
sterling. In 1636 the first advertisement of tea appeared in the *Mercurius
Politicus* as follows:

"The excellent Chinese beverage, recommended by all doctors,
which the Chinese call *teha* and other nations *tay* or *thé* is on sale in
the Café of the Sultana near the Royal Exchange."

Shortly afterwards tea was praised in Latin verses and found its
highest eulogy in a book by a Berlin author: "A cup of tea is a medium
for ensuring health and long life." The Dutch doctor, Bontekoe, who
later became the physician of the Prince Elector of Brandenburg, prescribed 100 to 200 cups a day. He himself drank tea day and night.

We here see a repetition of the conflict between praise and condemnation in the case of tea like that found in the history of other
excitants. Neither science nor experience can approve its condemnation. Besides the xanthine-complex caffeine, which is contained up
to 4.5 per cent, tea contains another xanthine, theophylline (theocin),
which is a dimethylxanthine. Both substances act synergetically, but
the latter, according to the observation of patients who have taken it
medicinally, is considerably more powerful. These circumstances were
instinctively taken into consideration long before the composition of
tea was known, by using far fewer tea leaves per cup than, for instance, coffee beans. There is no doubt that the abusive application of
concentrated infusions of tea is liable to call forth physical disorders
of a general nature in persons susceptible to its action, if only on account of the theophylline which, medicinally applied, is apt to give
rise to symptoms of convulsions. These are said to appear if more than
5 cups of a concentrated infusion of tea are consumed daily. A man
who from youth had become accustomed to drinking exaggerated quantities of tea and had reached a daily consumption of 30 cups suffered
from symptoms of anæmia, suffocation, and hallucinations. Men have
been known to drink 2 to 13 litres of tea daily, equaling 240 gr. of the
leaves. Facts of this kind are just as unsuitable a basis for judging the
good or bad properties of tea as are, for instance, the consequences of
daily excessive consumption of sodium bicarbonate or artificial fruit-
acid lemonades for a judgment of their properties. Even kitchen salt is
toxic in certain large doses.

The consequences which excessive amounts of tea are liable to produce may be ascertained in the Far East and in America where professional tea-tasters compare the value of the different kinds of tea by tasting infusions of it frequently two hundred times a day. Disorders of the gastric and intestinal functions, paleness or yellowness of the skin occur, and especially troubles of the nervous system: headache, hypochondria, weakness of memory, disturbances of the sight, and, it is said, also atrophy of the liver. It even appears that the abuse of tea by other persons is liable to give rise to hepatic disorders. Animal experiments have proved that the consequences of tea-poisoning frequently include modification of the liver and acute nephritis.

The consumption of large quantities of tea-leaves, which was once observed, also belongs to this group of aberrations. Half a pound of tea was consumed, giving rise to serious delirium.

A disagreeable state of excitation is also caused by the abuse which was and may still be customary in England of smoking cigarettes said to contain Haysan-tea. This abuse is principally practised by women, and one of these, a well-known novel-writer, smoked 20 to 30 such cigarettes daily during her work. Under these conditions one-quarter to three quarters of the caffeine originally contained in the tea, which is approximately 2 per cent, passes into the smoke, and is apt to reach the lungs. The consequences are trembling, general restlessness, palpitation of the heart, etc.

Setting aside these abusive applications of tea, there is hardly anything to be said against the habitual drinking of tea in moderation, even less than against coffee. Someone once stated that the drinking of strong coffee "certainly" promotes arteriosclerosis. This is "certainly" just as false as the report that swellings of the lymphatic glands, menstruation troubles, leucorrhœa, and diabetes are liable to occur. Excluding exaggerated doses and hypersensitive individuals it is true, on the contrary, that tea not only, like coffee, stimulates the digestion of amylaceous substances, and reinforces the absorption of gastric peptones and the casein of milk and cream, but also agreeably excites the central nervous system, which maintains or even slightly raises the normal degree of cerebral activity without resulting in a subjective impression of compulsion, i.e. an activity which cannot be mastered by the individual. These favourable effects are called forth even in cases where under normal circumstances fatigue would have diminished the active capacity. Besides giving rise to a certain kind of euphory, tea promotes the faculty of judgment and facilitates intellectual work, the maximum being reached after about forty minutes. Approximately 10 gr. of Pekoe tea increase the output of mental and muscular work by 10 per cent.

Animals also respond to tea by a state of excitation. On his expedition in Tibet, McGovern saw an ostler give a large vessel of strong tea to the weary horses. This method is in general use in such cases in Sikkim. The horses eagerly drink the tea and become nimble and active. A mule became so excited that it tried to run away and gambolled about like a young colt. The use of tea does not give rise to an imperative craving for its application or for an increase of the dose, as is the case with narcotics. Nevertheless such cases have been recorded in persons who exhibited other aberrations of cerebral life with respect to morbid desires.

The stimulating virtues of tea have in some countries, for instance England, introduced it into palace and cottage: "The cup that cheers but not inebriates."

And in Germany Uhland sang:

Ihr Saiten tönet sanft und leise,
Vom leichten Finger kaum geregt!
Ihr tönet zu des Zärtsten Preise,
Des Zärtsten, was die Erde hegt.
In Indiens mythischem Gebiete,
Wo Frühling ewig sich ernent,
O Tee, du selber eine Mythe,
Verlebst du deine Blütenzeit.[12]

Persons who are quite ignorant of the physiology of the human body know of tea and make use of its functional stimulation especially in order to augment physical and motor energy. The inhabitants of Tibet have no measure of time for short distances except the cup of tea. A member of the Mount Everest expedition asked a young peasant how far it was to the next village. He answered: "Three cups of tea." It was ascertained that three cups of tea is equal to 8 kilometres. This is, therefore, a measure of its stimulating and operative action. Tea would seem to be for the Tibetans the prime necessity of existence, and their main object of life to consist in obtaining as much as possible of the beverage. The Mongols are similar in this respect. They are also addicted to tea in the form of "tea-tiles," which are obtained by compression of tea-waste or of leaves of inferior quality and which in some cases serve as money. In order to give a proper consistency to these tiles it is said that they are kneaded together with a small amount of yak dung. A little piece is broken off and boiled in water, and after a certain time a lump of butter or suet is added to the resulting beverage. All tribes of this country come to Ta-tsien-lu (Gate of Tibet), the largest commercial center in the whole of Tibet, in order to load this tea on to thousands of yaks which transport it over snow and ice, through storms and the scorching heat of the sun, over passes and steppes to Lhasa, the seat of the Dalai Lama, and to Ladakh in Kashmir. Five million kilos are said to be transported in this way every year.

All the nomadic peoples of north-eastern Asia, the Tungus, Kamchadales, and Yakuts, love tea-drinking no less than the peoples of Central Asia, the Chinese, the Russians, and the English.

The large amounts consumed are furnished by extensive tea-plantations in the Far East which stretch from China to the Malay Archipelago and from the Chinese boundary to Ceylon. Although the export of tea to the various countries of the world fluctuates to a certain extent, the average annual amount consumed by the tea-drinking peoples is very nearly the same.

Table 10 shows the average quantity of tea consumed per head annually.[13]

TABLE 10. AVERAGE QUANTITY OF TEA CONSUMED ANNUALLY

England	2,500 gr.
Australia	2,500 gr.
United States	1,000 gr.
France	750 gr.
Holland	500 gr.
Russia	500 gr.
Scandinavia	250 gr.
Switzerland	150 gr.
Germany	100 gr.
Italy	30 gr.

Table 11 shows the fluctuations of the import of tea into Germany during the last few years. I am indebted to the German Statistical

Bureau (Statistischen Reichsamt) for this information.

TABLE 11. IMPORT OF TEA INTO GERMANY

COUNTRY OF ORIGIN	QUANTITY IN DOUBLE CENTNERS (100 KG.)								
	1911	1912	1913	1920	1921	1922	1923	1924	1925
British India	5167	5522	5910	2103	5805	4035	3220	7179	7896
Ceylon	3549	4043	4556	1069	4288	1892	2263	5762	7155
China	22006	24039	22884	1540	7083	5308	8367	12827	9770
Dutch E. Indies	5955	5804	7394	12050	36190	16702	10880	14683	16343
TOTAL	38124	41384	42903	17465	53771	28023	24782	40613	41518

The various peoples of the world prefer different caffeine beverages, but coffee and tea alone are really competitors. There are constant national preferences with respect to the latter. These preferences, the relatively high price, or the difficulty of obtaining the substances have given rise to the use of many substitutes. For coffee preparations of chicory, rye and especially barley, roasted pig-nuts, the seeds of the *carnauba* palm, acorns, figs, the seeds of *cassia occidentalis* known by the name of Fedegozo-Para-coffee, Mogdad coffee, or nigger-coffee, the seeds of *hibiscus sabdariffa* used by the people of Emin Pasha, the seeds of *gymnocladus dioeca* (Kentucky coffee), lupins, etc., are used. The number of plants used as substitutes for genuine tea is extremely large. I am aware of some two hundred, among them the following: *vaccinium uliginosum* (Batum tea), *vaccinium myrtillus* (Caucasian tea), *angrœcum fragrans* (Faham tea, Bourbon tea), *cyclopia genistoides* (Cape or Bush tea), which contains just as little caffeine as the nigger-coffee cited above, *ledum latifolium* (Labrador or James tea), *ledum palustre*, *gaultheria procumbens* (Mountain tea or Canadian tea), *ceanothus americanus* (New Jersey tea), *chenopodium ambrosioides* (Mexico tea), *monarda didyma* (Oswego or Pennsylvania tea), *capraria biflora* (West Indian tea), *alstonia theœformis* (Bogota tea), *stachytarpheta* (Brazilian tea), *erva cidreira*, *psoralea glandulosa* (Jesuits' tea), *helichrysum serpyllifolium* (Hottentot tea), *epilobium hirsutum* (Kapporia tea, Copnic tea, Iwan tea), *lithospermum officinale* (Bohemian or Croatian tea), *salvia officinalis*, various Veronicas, Verbascum, *rubus arcticus*, *dryas octopetala*, *saxifraga crassifolia*, *lepidium ruderale* (Homeriana tea), the nettle plant in Tibet, etc.

All these plants and many others used as substitutes for tea have nothing in common with that substance. In the most favourable case they contain some essential oil which is far from possessing the properties which act on the brain like the purine compounds caffeine, theobromine, etc. Their value may be likened to that of a wooden leg in comparison with a healthy leg.

I look upon coffee, tea, or other stimulating substances from which the active principles have been chemically removed in the same light. They are castrated products which have lost their capability of creating energy.

THE KOLA NUT

History, Origin, Distribution

The population of the vast territory of the Sudan between the Atlantic Ocean and the source of the Nile crave for a substance which supplies them in everyday life with a slight feeling of stimulation and temporarily augments physical capacity. The kola nut is the drug which satisfies these desires. Its stimulating effects on physical activity have endowed it with a considerable market value, and have not prevented it from penetrating far into the north across the Sahara up to Fezzan. Mohammedans, "pagans," and others love the kola nut and make great sacrifices in order to procure it.

This nut plays an important part in the social life and commercial relations of these peoples. Much trouble is taken in order to obtain the drug. The Haussa, for instance, organize long caravan-journeys for this purpose to the country of the Ashanti, and their arrival is an important event for the latter. Those who have no money to buy the drug beg. Rich people ingratiate themselves by distributing nuts or pieces of nuts. The inhabitant of Kano in northern Nigeria does not hesitate to sell his horse or his best slave, his two most important possessions, in order to enjoy his favourite pastime. Indeed, it is not rare for a poor man to seize an already half-masticated piece of another person's nut and to continue chewing it.

The physical effects of kola must evidently be very considerable, or it would not be so highly esteemed. The habit of chewing it cannot alone be regarded as sufficient explanation. That is why the first

discovery of kola, as in many other cases of a similar kind, has been
explained by a divine legend:

> One day when the Creator was on earth observing the sons of men
> and busy among them, he put aside a piece of the kola nut which he
> was chewing and forgot to take it with him when he went away
> again. A man saw this and seized the dainty morsel. His wife tried
> to prevent him from tasting the food of God. The man, however,
> placed it in his mouth and found that it tasted good. While he was
> still chewing the Creator returned, sought the forgotten piece of
> kola, and saw how the man tried to swallow it. He quickly grasped
> at his throat and forced him to return the fruit. Since that time
> there can be seen in the throat of man the 'Adam's apple,' the trace
> of the pressure of the fingers of God.

If, leaving the intervention of the Creator out of the question, we
seek the epoch in which the first knowledge of this vegetable product
was obtained, we encounter the first reports of the fruit in the writings
of El Ghafeky, a learned Spanish physician, who lived in the twelfth
century, and those of the botanist, Ebn El-Baithar, who lived in the
thirteenth. The former's description of the fruit may apply to the kola-
tree, but his characterization of the seeds does not agree so well.[14] We
do not come across the name *kola* until the latter part of the sixteenth
century, when it is mentioned by travellers and explorers, for instance
Carolus Clusius, Duarte Barbos, Dapper, etc.

The tree which furnishes the kola nut is *sterculia* or *cola acuminata*.[15]
It is about 15 to 20 metres in height and has a straight smooth trunk.
Each female blossom has five carpels which after fecundation become
follicles arranged star-fashion. Each follicle may reach 15 cm. in length
and contains up to eight seeds which are approximately 4 cm. in length
and 3 cm. thick, similar to horse chestnuts, light or dark red in colour
and emitting an odour similar to freshly-cut Maréchal Niel roses. These
seeds are the kola nuts. There are also spurious kola nuts which are
white and very bitter and originate from a tree called *garcinia cola*.
These latter do not contain an alkaloid like the genuine kola nuts.
Many other seeds similar to kola nuts, but inactive, have appeared on
the market, and probably also in preparations of kola, such as the seeds
of *cola supfiana* (Avatimeko kola nut), *dimorphandra mora* (West Indian kola nut), *pentedesma butyracea*, etc.

The genuine kola nut has various names: Goro, Guru, Ombene, Nangue, Biche, Makatso, Gonja, etc. The tree which produces them grows wild and is also cultivated on the west coast of Africa from Sierra Leone and Liberia up to the lower part of the Congo and Guinea, from 10° north latitude to 5° south latitude, most frequently out of the reach of the ocean winds, and in a wild state mainly in Futa Jallon, on the banks of the Rio Nuñez, and in Ashantiland. It occurs in the interior as far as the mountain ridge to the south of the Mandingo territories. It does not grow on the Mandigo Plain. In the hinterland of Lagos, for instance near Ikere, there are even kola forests. The cultivation of the tree has been brought to a state of perfection by the natives. It grows in the south of Benue in Adamawa and the nuts are brought to Bornu. The plant also occurs in Monbuttuland and farther to the north in a wild state.

The kola-tree has been transported from Africa to India, the Seychelles, Ceylon, Damaraland, Dominica, Mauritius, Sydney, Zanzibar, Guadeloupe, Cayenne, and Cochin China. After nine or ten years one tree supplies approximately 30 kg. of dry nuts.

In this immense zone of Africa the kola nut is utilized in some places, by the Monbutto and the Niam-Niam for example, only occasionally, and in Wadai it was only used by the king, who obtained it from Bornu. The kola nut is known to the Arabs as "Sudan coffee," and it is also highly valued by the non-Arabic inhabitants of Africa, such as the Ashantis, the Wute in the Cameroons, the negroes of the Congo, and the tribes in the neighbourhood of and to the west of Albert-Edward-Nyanza. Many men are engaged in the commerce and transport of this relatively precious substance. From the coast of West Africa, from Futa Jallon, Sankaran, Kuranko, between the rivers Rio Grande in Portuguese Guinea and St. Paul in Liberia, the nuts were formerly transported (and it is not likely that great changes have taken place in the meantime) in basket-loads of 3,500 nuts on the heads of male and female slaves to the markets of Kankan, Timé, Tengrela, Maninian, and Sambatiguilla, by Mandingo merchants mainly in exchange for salt. Farther to the south there are also markets in Odienné, Kani, Siana, and Sakhala, where the kola agents, the Mandé-Diula, fix the prices. There they are exchanged for cotton and salt (the latter coming from the north of the Sahara, i.e. Timbuctu and Arawan) by merchants from Segu and Jenne. The cotton which serves as an object of exchange is produced by the Bambara, who inhabit the territory between the upper Senegal and the Niger. After marches which frequently last for months, the nuts, which often have to be repacked, are transported on the Niger to Timbuctu. The nuts of the Ashanti country and the Mohammedan state of Salaga, which is a kind of commercial metropolis, are also bartered in the north. Mossi and Haussa merchants transport the nuts to Sinder, Timbuctu, etc., or to Sokoto, Katsena, Kano, and Bornu, from whence they are delivered via Kuka on Lake Chad in a northern direction and also by way of the desert and in the south-east via Shari to Bagirmi. Kola nut bearers also take other routes to the south and the east through Nigeria and the Cameroons in the direction of the Congo, through forests, over rivers and mountains, to enable the population to make use of the drug. From Sierra Leone whole deck-loads of nuts with Mandingos as deck-passengers go by boat to the ports of Senegambia.

The kola nut of Sakala is the largest and most expensive known. It is delivered for the greater part to Jenne and Timbuctu. The nuts from Khani, Siana, and Touté are of middle size, and are especially in demand when of a red colour. A very small red nut, the kola from Maninian, can be bought in Jenne and Tiomakandugu. These nuts, like every eagerly desired substance which modifies cerebral activity, are fairly expensive. Everything, even slaves, can be bought with nuts. At times one nut costs in Gorea three to five pence; on the banks of the Niger four shillings had to be paid for one nut, and if money were short a slave could be bought for a few nuts. If the kola nut were exclusively used as a means to supply energy or pleasurable sensations it would not attain such high prices. It is, however, like the betel nut, so important a symbol in the various events of everyday life that the demand for it and its consumption are considerably increased. A proposal of marriage is accompanied by a gift of white kola; a refusal by red nuts. Kola must not be lacking from the dowry. Oaths are sworn on the kola nut, friendships or hostilities are symbolized by kola and some nuts are even buried with the dead.

Effects of Kola

As a rule pieces of the fresh nut are chewed. The taste is at first bitter and afterwards sweet. The powder of the dried nut is also consumed and occasionally, e.g. by the Bagunda, the Banalya, and on the banks of the Lulua and the Aruwimi, a beverage is prepared from the dried nuts which is imbibed with the aid of a reed-cane. The effects are very similar to those of other substances which contain caffeine. In this case sleep is dispensed thanks to the excitation of the brain due to kola. The feeling of hunger does not appear in its habitual strength after consumption of kola and, if felt beforehand, is thereby considerably diminished. These statements are not only the result of experiences in Africa but also of observations during strenuous Alpine tours in Europe. An increase of muscular energy and resistance without a feeling of fatigue is even more marked. Physical strength is augmented without the intervention of the will. During long marches or difficult climbs in the mountains it is most evident that movement is facilitated and that the increased output of the muscles, even if it is hot, is not accompanied by exhaustion. These effects have been very frequently experienced not only under the influence of the pure drug but also after consumption of kola biscuits or other preparations from it.

Experiments carried out on horses which were fed solely on kola during their labours proved that the output of work increased. Thorough investigations of general metabolism in animals and in man have revealed the fact that the combustion of carbohydrates and fat is augmented under the influence of kola, but that of nitrogenous substances, both urea and the nitrogenous bodies in general, and of phosphates is very markedly reduced. Consequently the kola nut may be regarded as an economizer of the orgnaism not only with respect to the muscular but also to the nervous system.

It has repeatedly been stated that kola, like other caffeine substances, acts as a stimulant in the sexual sphere. According to the opinion of the inhabitants of Africa it has an aphrodisiac effect on men and promotes conception in women. In this general form this supposition is not correct; it may be, however, that kola acts in some individual cases in the manner indicated.

Personal disposition naturally exercises a great influence on the effects of kola, especially if it is taken in large quantities, as in every case where the chemical properties of a substance react on the chemistry of the organism. It may happen, as I have heard from the experience of Count Goetzen himself, that a state of general weakness and prostration sets in. In the case of another, a vigorous and strong man, serious cephalic congestion, trembling and insomnia appeared a few hours after ingestion of two fresh nuts.

Exhaustive research work has been carried out in order to ascertain whether caffeine is the only active principle in kola or whether other substances contained in the nut are also of biological importance. Comparative investigations of the metabolism in animals seem to prove that powdered kola nut has a more powerful effect than a corresponding quantity of pure caffeine.

There is no doubt that the kola nut is chemically more complex than the other vegetable products which contain caffeine. An essential oil with a strong aromatic taste is very probably also active in producing the effects described. Women who were engaged in the work of cutting up the nuts into small pieces at first became very excited and then suffered from insomnia through the action of the odour of the essential oil. However it is caffeine which endows kola with its characteristic action. It is contained in the drug up to 2 per cent. It may be that the theobromine which occurs to a slight extent in the nut is also active as an excitant. It has not been ascertained in spite of many experiments whether other substances co-operate with the caffeine. In fresh kola nuts there is a crystalline phenolic principle belonging to the group of tannins, kolatin,[16] which is present from 0.3 to 0.4 per cent in unstable combination with the caffeine. Hot water dissociates the complex. Under certain circumstances kolatin can be oxidized into insoluble kola-red. In nuts which are dried in the usual manner the kolatin disappears, but it can be preserved by sterilization. The dark colour which appears during the process of exsiccation of the nuts is due to the decomposition of an oxydase which is present in the nut.

The conclusion at which we arrive after taking the chemical results into consideration is that from a pharmacological point of view the opinion which ascribes the principal part in the action of kola to caffeine should not be altered, even if further research should throw light on the interdependence of the various components of the nut and even if the crystallized kolatin is considered to be active. For this reason neither kola-red and the other substances cited above nor the enzymes, including kola-lipase, are of importance in the total effect. It is said that there exists a kind of antagonism between kolatin and caffeine whereby the former produes no increase of muscular work and no cerebral excitation. Even if this were true, caffeine would maintain its qualitatively and quantitatively predominant position in the action of kola, as may be ascertained in animals and man after the ingestion of the fresh nut. I myself have been able to make these observations with the fresh nuts which I have frequently obtained from Georg Schwinfurth.

ILEX PARAGUAYENSIS: MATÉ

About one hundred years ago Aimé Bonpland, the great naturalist and philanthropist, the friend and travelling-companion of Alexander von Humboldt, set out on a new expedition. Loaded with honours and highly esteemed by Napoleon and the Empress Josephine, he left France after the fall of the Empire and the death of the Empress, whose disease he had as a medical man correctly diagnosed. The greatest honours offered to him were not able to hold him back. After having worked for some time in Buenos Aires he continued his explorations, reaching Paranà and the ancient Jesuit missions in the disputed territory between Paraguay and the Argentine. He wrote to the dictator Francia that he intended devoting himself to the cultivation of maté with the aid of Indians whom he had enrolled. The suspicious and inexorably cruel dictator had him and his family attacked by night. Bonpland himself was wounded and carried off in chains. He spent nearly ten years in prison and earned his livelihood by the preparation of pharmaceutical products. But even during this period of utter poverty he devoted himself as a physician to the well-being of the sick. In spite of all the efforts of the French Government and of the Emperor Dom Pedro I, he was not set free until 1830, and died at the age of eighty on his ranch in Uruguay. He had established a large maté plantation in Candelaria.

These distant events are recalled when we attempt to describe maté, a caffeine plant which is extensively employed by all social classes in a large section of humanity amounting to approximately 15 million people in the south of Brazil, the La Plata States, Chile, Bolivia, part of Peru, and the Argentine.

In the virgin forests of Paraguay, which are as large as whole European kingdoms, from the savage Matto Grosso, still in a primeval state, to the basin of the immense Paranà with its numerous tributary streams, there still exist immense forests of *Ilex paraguayensis*, an evergreen tree occurring invarious forms. This territory extends from 18° to 30° south latitude at a height of approximately 500 metres above sea-level in the Brazilian states of Paranà, Santa Caterina, and Rio Grande do Sul, as well as over some parts of the states of São Paulo and Minas Gerães. The tree reaches a height of 4 to 8 or even 12 metres. It is called simply yerba, or in Brazil maté, herva maté, congonha; in the Argentine yerba maté, congoin, and in Paraguay caaguaza. The leaves and young branches are used for an infusion similar to tea. Indians and half-castes scour the forests, where they erect huts covered with palm-leaves or straw and level a part of the earth for the drying of the leaves. They cut off with their large knives the tops of the branches with the leaves. The material is partly dried, and in order to prevent it from turning black it is passed through flames and then dried on trellis-work over an open fire for three to four days. It is then reduced to small pieces with wooden clubs or crushed to a crude powder in the forest. In larger works a cylinder fitted with teeth is rolled over the maté on the barn floor with the aid of a horse and a kind of capstan; the maté is then reduced to a fine powder in stamping mills.

Various kinds of preparations of maté are to be found in commerce; the young leaves which are dried in the sun and soon lose their aroma (caa-kuy), elder leaves which have been carefully separated from the branches (caa-mirim), and the product prepared from the leaves and the stems (caa-guaza). The caffeine content of the unroasted leaves reaches 1.7 per cent and the torrefied product 0.6 per cent. Maté moreover contains a small amount of essential oil and a tannin which is identical with caffeo-tannic acid.[17]

It is probable that maté was prepared in ancient times in a still simpler manner. The origin of its use is quite unknown; it is buried with the ancestors of the peoples of that part of the world. Our ignorance of its history is as great as in the case of most of the other substances described in this work. It is surprising that here also an analogy exists between the primitive preparation of maté and that of coffee-beans and tea-leaves. In the case of all three plants a kind of torrefaction process is carried out which serves as a preservative and at the same time develops the aroma. When the Europeans arrived in America they not only discovered the method of preparation of maté but also its employment as a means of exchange between the Indians.

At the present day the Gaucho in the Pampa, the Caboclo in the virgin forest, the solitary horseman and the inhabitant of the city drink the infusion of the prepared leaves with the same relish. In the Argentine the annual consumption per head of the inhabitants amounts to approximately 6 kilos, whereas only 1 kilo of tea and 250 gr. of coffee are consumed. Uruguay imports 6 million kilos annually, mainly from Brazil. This quantity is said to correspond to 10 kilos per head of the inhabitants per annum.

Maté is drunk several times a day. A hollow gourd as large as a man's fist, in the form of a bottle, serves as a receptable, which among the rich is decorated with gold or silver. Two spoonfuls of maté are placed in this cup and moistened with a little cold water. Two or three minutes later boiling water is added. After approximately the same lapse of time the beverage is ready to be taken. For this purpose a pipe made of precious metal or of tin or a vegetable fibre, to the lower extremity of which a small spherical sieve is attached, is plunged into the beverage. The liquid is sucked in by means of this "bombilla." The drink has a peculiar aroma to which one soon becomes accustomed and an agreeable and mild taste.

Its action differs only slightly from that of the other caffeine beverages. Besides diminishing the feeling of thirst on long marches or when the heat of the sun renders it intolerable, it acts as a tonic for the nerves without any disagreeable by-effects and without suppressing the desire to sleep. Physical energy is also augmented. The working capacity of the muscles is considerably increased without giving rise to an impression of compulsion. A stimulation of the renal functions is, moreover, a constant property of all substances containing purines.

Maté as a beverage has no disagreeable by-effects. It has nevertheless been stated by a person who probably had a very weak stomach that large doses gave rise to nausea, sleepiness and feebleness in the legs. But there are certainly not many members of the human race who are so sensitive.

ILEX CASSINE

In 1562 Captain Laudonnière, who was exploring the coast of Florida at the request of Admiral Coligny and with the approval of King

Charles IX of France in order to find a new home for the French Protestants, discovered that the natives consumed a beverage which they called cassine. Shortly before this time the Conquistadores Narvaez and Cabeza de Vaca had made the same discovery. Laudonnière was presented with some basketfuls of the plant with which this beverage was prepared. The plant served as a commodity of exchange among the Indians of the western parts. Who can tell how long the drug had been in use before Europeans set foot in the country? Perhaps it was employed even in prehistoric days at a time when man had recourse to any vegetable in order to vary the primitive conditions of his existence. The properties of plants were not ascertained by divination, but by experiment. Thousands must have met their death in the course of these experiments before others learnt how to distinguish between the useful and the useless, the harmful and the harmless.

This is probably the way in which the stimulating properties of ilex cassine (*ilex vomitoria, i. dahoon, i. religiosa, yaupon, yopon*) were discovered. It is a shrub or small tree 3 to 6 metres in height which grows in a wild state, especially in the woody coastal regions of North and South Carolina, Georgia, and Florida, and it also occurs near the lower course of the Mississippi, in Texas, and near the Colorado valley.

The Indians of the above-named territories used to employ the plant far more extensively than, for instance, the Creek Indians do at the present day when celebrating religious festivals. The leaves and young branches are used in a fresh state or dried and roasted in flat receptacles for the preparation of the beverage. The sharp and bitter "black drink" is taken during two or three days in assemblies from which women and children are excluded. Repeated vomiting is the result. The Indians alternately drink and vomit until the body is "cleansed" and they feel fit for new enterprises. These effects are accompanied by irritations of the intestines and the kidneys.[18]

In addition to an essential oil, caffeine from 0.3 to 1.6 per cent and a tannic acid have been ascertained in the leaves. There is so much caffeine in the plant that it has recently been recommended for the extraction of the drug. In all likelihood such large quantities of concentrated infusions of the plant are imbibed that the exciting action of the alkaloid becomes manifest not only in the brian but also in other organs depending upon its action, for instance, the kidneys, in a very marked form. It is stated, moreover, that substances are added which irritate the gastric mucus to such an extent that vomiting is produced, to which the Indians attribute a special significance.

The most important active element in ilex cassine is caffeine.

According to the observations of Karsten a hitherto unknown species of Ilex is used by the Jibáros and Canelos Indians as an aqueous infusion and as a mouth-wash under the name of *guayusa*. The leaves of the guayusa-tree, which grows everywhere in eastern Ecuador, supply an aromatic beverage which is prepared only by the men but is drunk by the women also. Concentrated infusion gives rise to vomiting as in the case of ilex cassine. This cleansing of the stomach seems to be greatly desired. Guayusa is also considered a magic beverage which strengthens the body for hunting expeditions.

PASTA GUARANA

Our attention is again drawn to the insoluble riddle of the first discovery of the properties of a substance in the case of Pasta Guarana. How did the savage tribes scattered in the basin of the Amazon, of the Madeira and the Tapajoz, or above the equator between the Magdalena and the Orinoco discover one day long ago that a plant of the Sapindaceae family could be consumed as a tonic agent on account of its caffeine content? How was the dry, husk-like and in no way remarkable fruit of that climbing creeper, *paullinia sorbilis (paullinia cupana)* distinguished with respect to its caffeine content from the fruits of all the other numerous species of *paullinia* that grow in those parts? Perhaps an inhabitant of the forests, weary and dying of hunger after an unsuccessful hunting expedition, had recourse to the seeds, chewed them, and soon experienced a feeling of comfort, refreshment, and lessened hunger. These are questions which will never be answered.

At the present time, as in days of yore, the Maués and Mundurukús of the lower and middle Tapajoz collect in October the completely ripe dark-brown seeds which are contained in pear-like capsules terminating in a short point. They scrape or grind them and knead the resulting powder on heated slabs with water to a paste. After adding a few whole seeds the substance is rolled into cylinders approximately 12 to 30 cm. long and up to 5 cm. thick, which if dried in smoke keep for many years. Amylaceous substances are regularly added to this plastic mass, such as mandioca starch and cocoa powder. This is the origin of Guarana Paste[19] with the aid of which the Indians prepare a beverage, *aqua branca*, i.e. white water, which is an article of export to Bolivia, Matto Grosso, etc. The canoes which in spite of the numerous cataracts and rapids come from Matto Grosso down the Arinos and Tapajoz loaded with ipecacuanha and hides take in at Santarem on the Amazon, which is an imoprtant commercial centre for the traffic in guarana, a valuable return freight of guarana lumps. In the same way the large boats on the Madeira always transport a certain quantity of the drug to Bolivia, for in Cuyabá as well as in Santa Cruz de la Sierra and Cochabamba there are many persons who cannot live without guarana, and would rather fast than forbear drinking the beverage. In these parts the price of guarana is approximately ten times as high as it is in the countries of origin inhabited by the Maués and the Mundurukús. Many Bolivians take the beverage soon after sunrise immediately on awakening and cannot carry out their day's work without it. The tribes occupied with its preparation do not consume it to a considerable extent.

Guarana paste is as hard as stone, as brown as chocolate, and has a slightly bitter taste. In the preparation of the beverage it is scraped as fine as possible with a grater or the hard palate of a fish, the pirarucú (*sudis gigas*). Sugar is then added and one teaspoonful of the powder is drunk cold, with a glass of water. Its taste reminded me of almonds or cocoa. According to the observations of Crevaux, the Piapoko, who inhabit the territory between the Magdalena and the Orinoco, scrape the quarter of an unripe fruite approximately 12 mm. long, called *cupanna*, and drink it with water.

As the seeds contain 4 to 5 per cent caffeine, and the guarana paste may contain the same amount, it will be understood that a beverage with exciting properties prepared from this drug will be highly appreciated and eagerly desired. Naturally, it is occasionally applied to abuse, and the symptoms of increased nervous excitability which arise are the same as in the case of coffee and tea.

COCOA

In 1528, Hernando Cortez returned to Spain bringing as a result of his expedition the news of the conquest of Mexico and the knowledge of cocoa and its use. The importance which he himself attributed to the plant is clearly shown in a letter to the Emperor Charles V, in which he describes the plantations of the fruit-supplying tree: "On the lands of one farm two thousand trees have been planted; the fruits are similar to almonds and are sold in a powdered state."

How long have the Mexicans utilized the seeds for general consumption? The answer is "always," in the same sense and to the same extent as in all other substances of this kind. The Spaniards found the beans in use as small coin in commercial traffic in Mexico, rates and taxes were paid with theobroma seeds. The whole population consumed the preparation habitually. Fifty vessels of aromatic chocolate were prepared daily for the Emperor Montezuma. It had a consistency similar to honey, was served in golden goblets, and eaten with spoons of gold or decorated tortoise-shell. Chocolate early found its way from Mexico to Spain in the form of tablets or slabs and soon became popular. It did not reach other countries till many years later. In Flanders and Italy it did not appear before 1606. Antonio Colmenero reported in 1631, that the number of cocoa-users in these countries was very considerable. The complicated Mexican mode of preparing the beverage, which he described, was soon simplified, and only sugar or honey, vanilla, and cinnamon was added to the cocoa. In the year 1650, chocolate was introduced into France and England.

Its triumphant conquest of the rest of the world soon took place, but not without its meeting exaggerated praise and censure. Some considered the beverage as a vital necessity:

Ambrosia est Superum potus, cocolata virorum:
Haec hominum vitam protrahit, illa deum.

The beverage of the Gods was Ambrosia; that of man is chocolate.
Both increase the length of life in a prodigious manner.

A poet once went thus far in his eulogy, and Linnæus called the tree which supplies the cocoa bean *theobroma cacao*, i.e. cocoa, the food of the gods. On the other hand, Benzoni at the end of the sixteenth century thought chocolate more fit for pigs than for men, and the great botanist Lécluse was of the same opinion: *Porcorum eaverius colluvies quam hominum potio.* It is not possible to discuss questions of individual taste. The opinion of some persons does not prevent a substance like cocoa from exercising its attractive powers on human appreciation and desire. The consumption of chocolate only diminished in the time of Federick II because criminals used it as a vehicle of poison. Apart from this, the use of cocoa has increased considerably during recent centuries, especially in the last few decades. Its progress is more rapid than that of tea or coffee. Whereas the consumption of tea in Germany has increased three and a half times in the last thirty years, that of cocoa increased twelve times up to 1914. In 1908, 0.52 kilogramme, and in 1912 0.81 kilogrammes of cocoa was imported per head of the population.

While in days of old cocoa was the favourite beverage of the Spanish-American peoples only, from Mexico to Chile, without excepting those who prepare excellent coffee, e.g. the inhabitants of Guatemala and Costa Rica, it is at the present day increasingly appreciated in other countries. Nevertheless it is consumed to the greatest extent by the Spaniards and Portuguese, whose consumption equals 1 kilogramme per head of the population.

Theobroma cacao is a tree 6 to 12 metres in height; it originates in the hot parts of America (Mexico, Guatemala, Guiana, Venezuela, Colombia, Ecuador, etc.), and is cultivated in Asia (Java, the Philippines, etc.), in Africa (Togo, Cameroon, East Africa, Bourbon), and in the Greater and Lesser Antilles. It produces seeds in the form of beans of a bitter taste which are either left to a kind of fermentation in pits in the earth for a few days or are dried in the sun and then worked up.

The components of the raw and peeled beans are mainly characterized by 2 per cent theobromine, fatty matter more than 50 per cent, starch up to 15 per cent, and a total amount of nitrogen of 16 per cent.

Before human consumption the seeds are subjected to several processes, such as roasting with supercharged steam at a temperature of 130°C in order to remove the fatty matter. Nevertheless cocoa powder generally still contains about 13 to 38 per cent fat. Foreign substances are largely added to the commercial varieties, but the ordinary composition of cocoa indicates its nourishing qualities.

May cocoa be regarded as having other properties than those of a valuable foodstuff? Its theobromine is accompanied by small quantities of caffeine. Theobromine is dimethylxanthine, caffeine is trimethylxanthine. Both belong to the group of purines, several of which are products of the chemical processes of the human organism. According to my interpretation these purines (whether methylated or not) are not only produts but also active substances. I think they are excitants for certain functions of the organism, among others those of the ductless glands, even if they are only produced in minute quantities in the body. The stimulating effects of cocoa increase with its theobromine content. The stimulating action of theobromine is doubtless far inferior to that of caffeine, but it exists, although less evident than that of the latter. Individual differences in the energy of the effects may naturally be ascertained not only after ingestion of theobromine but also after consumption of cocoa. There are extremely sensitive persons who experience cardiac and visual disturbances, as well as gastric disorders, even after the consumption of chocolate.

The stimulating effects of cocoa have been proved by direct experiment with a daily consumption fo 25 to 30 gr. Single doses of 25 gr. also gave rise to disagreeable toxic symptoms such as trembling, headaches, acceleration of the pulse, etc. In isolated cases these deviations from the normal effects have been observed after consumption of chocolate. It cannot be ascertained to what extent foreign additions to the cocoa substance are responsible for these effects.

TOBACCO

Historical and General Information

There are many ways of classifying and distinguishing the peoples of the world. They might be enumerated according to profession, rank, belief, nationality, political opinion, temperament, physical and mental qualities, and so on. The use of tobacco, however, permits us to reduce these categories to two: smokers and non-smokers. More than that, this classification has a practical importance in everyday life. Those who want to indulge in the habit of smoking must travel in separate compartments. There are smoking and nonsmoking compartments. The smoker is obliged to refrain from his desire when entering a place where an atmosphere of dignity reigns: one does not smoke in church, or in the law-courts, nor when entering the houses of people one does not know very well.

It is not tobacco as such but the mode of its application which has placed this substance in a class by itself. For the discreet, snuffing or chewing of tobacco is not in the least subject to social restrictions, though it is just as much a form of nicotinism as smoking. In former times, however, the smoking of tobacco in public, even where the sanctity of the locality or respect of persons did not arise, was considered an infringement of social morality and even punished. In Prussia the prohibition of smoking in the street was not abolished till the year 1848.

The use of tobacco has been subjected to the common lot of all similar substances. Hated and beloved by man, its destiny was ruled by the changes of the ages and the progress of civilization. These vicissitudes were perhaps more marked in the case of tobacco than in that of the other substances. At the present day its irresistible penetration among the habits of both the primitive and highly civilized peoples of the earth is continually increasing, and can only be compared to that of alcohol; it even surpasses the latter, since the religious motives which in the Orient excluded alcohol as an intoxicating substance do not apply.

On October 12, 1492, Christopher Columbus dropped anchor at Guanahani, one of the Bahama Islands. On October 29 he drew near Cuba and on November 2 he sent two Spaniards on an expedition from which they returned on November 6. They reported that they had met many men and women who held in their hands a piece of burning charcoal which they maintained with the aid of odoriferous herbs. These consisted of dry herbs wrapped up in a large dry leaf; they were like the small muskets with which Spanish children play at Whitsun. They were lighted at one end and the people sucked at the other and drank the smoke, as it were, by inhaling it. This rendered them somnolent and intoxicated, but apparently inhibited the experience of fatigue. The people call these kinds of muskets "tabacos." De las Casas, the Bishop of Chiapas, who published the letters of Columbus in which this description is contained, states: "I know of Spaniards who imitate this custom, and when I reprimanded the savage practice, they answered that it was not in their power to refrain from indulging in the habit. Although the Spaniards were extremely surprised by this peculiar custom, on experimenting with it themselves they soon obtained such pleasure that they began to imitate the savage example." In this way one of the most powerful motives which influence man and human events, the instinct of imitation, vindicated itself. Very soon detailed descriptions of the various means of tobacco-smoking were forthcoming. Only four years later the hermit Romano Pane, whom Columbus after his second voyage left on Hispaniola (Haiti) in order to convert the natives, and who learnt their language and customs, described the habit of inhaling the fumes with the aid of a forked pipe which was inserted into the nostrils and held over the smoking tobacco which was glowing on charcoal. He also described the properties of this smoke, which intoxicated the smokers and rendered him sleepy. Other documents of this period tell us that those who were under the influence of tobacco-smoke regarded their sensations and dreams as supernatural and therefore considered the plant sacred. We may, however, state at once that in the mode of smoking above indicated the narcotic effects accompanied by diminished consciousness are mainly due to the carbon monoxide of the burning charcoal which is inhaled together with the tobacco fumes.

Heavy work in the mines, famine, and the cruelty of the Spaniards reduced the number of Indians, which was estimated at three million, in a few decades to 20,000. The abominable import of negroes from Africa commenced at this time. The Christian Genoese were responsible for it. Pope Leo X declared it permissible because the negroes, not being Christians, were not suited to be at liberty, and the knowledge of the Gospel compensated them for their loss of freedom. These negroes soon became accustomed to tobacco and, according to the observations of Oviedo y Valdes in 1513, cultivated the plant on their masters' plantations.

Bishop de las Casas, who protested against this kidnapping and the other misdeeds of the Christians, experienced the same impressions as Columbus on seeing the Indians smoking. The use of tobacco (*petuna*) was known in all the islands of the Antilles and the neighboring continent at the time of Columbus' voyages. The Aztecs and Toltecs in Mexico smoked tobacco in pipes finely painted and gilt or made of burnt clay. The herb, which was consecrated to the goddess Cihuacoatl, was called ye (yetl). In the years 1512 to 1535 this custom was also practised in Central America, Yucatan, Darien, Panama, and Brazil, but not by all the tribes. It was unknown on the banks of the La Plata, in Prana and Paraguay, and in the countries of the west coast, Quito, Peru, and Chile. In 1512, at the time when Ponce de Leon

discovered Florida, Indians and in 1535 Canadians, were observed to
be addicted to smoking tobacco (*upawoc*).

Excavations made during the last century in several of the United
States of America which have revealed tobacco pipes, seem to prove
that the use of tobacco also extended to other parts of America. This
is not surprising, for commerce and trade between one people and
another and migration of whole races has taken place as long as mankind has existed. The final result has been the extension of the use of
tobacco to the most distant parts of the world, and there is no language, however poor in words it may be, without an expression for
tobacco, just as there exist everywhere words for bread, water, and
death.

The whole of Asia from the coast of the Mediterranean to the
Polar Sea and eastward to the Pacific Ocean, with its world of islands,
extending beyond the Torres Straits to Australia, represents an enormous territory where tobacco is smoked, and occasionally snuffed or
chewed, frequently with such avidity that we arrive at the conclusion
that the nicotine habit is an integral part of the lives of the inhabitants. In the south of Nias the first greeting is usually: "*Faniso Toca'!*"
"*Faniso sabe'e,*" i.e. "Tobacco, sir, strong tobacco," and then: "We die,
sir, if we have no tobacco."

Tobacco is also very extensively employed over the whole of
America, from the boundary of the Polar Sea, including Greenland,
to Tierra del Fuego, and in Europe it is also used to a great extent;
likewise in Africa from the Straits of Gibraltar to the Cape of Good
Hope and from the western to the eastern coast. Primitive races and
highly refined Europeans are equally prone to its use; just as are the
Wawira, the Pygmy tribes of the majestic forests of Africa, the primitive Bushman of the vast Kalahari desert, the man whose country is
the sun-parched plains of the Sahara, the Eskimo, who is indifferent
to eternal snow, frost, and icy tempests because his physical organism
represents the finest example of teleological adaptation, or the South
Sea islander who lives in the tropical splendor and primitive super-
abundance of the fertility of nature.

On the other hand the number of tobaccophobes, those who oppose tobacco in Europe and other countries, is hardly worth mention-
ing. The Parsis for instance, who look upon fire as the Almighty and
the universal purifying element, refrain for this reason from profaning

it by smoking. The Sikhs in India, the religious sect of the Semeskes in the valley of Chikoi on the way from Kyashta to Urga, the Modammedan Tungus or the Russian sect of the Kirshaks, who live in the Altai between Southern Siberia and Mongolia and, although drinkers of spirits, have renounced tobacco, the monks in the cloisters of Central Korea, strictly observant Moors, the Rif people who only snuff, all these refrain from smoking tobacco. Some Abyssinian Christians seek to distinguish themselves from Mohammedans by renouncing tobacco, and among some tribes of the Sinai Peninsula trading in and possession of tobacco are said to be severely punished. The Senüssi of the Libyan desert, the inhabitants of some islands of the Pacific Ocean, for instance the Purdy Island near the Admiralty Islands, and the natives of New Hanover do not smoke. Nevertheless, the descendants of all these tribes and sects will one day make the close acquaintance of tobacco in the form of smoke or powder as an excitant for their mucous membrane. Without taking these relatively unimportant exceptions into consideration it will be found that tobacco is used over the whole world, whether man is at work or at rest, during his daily struggle for the means of existence or when peacefully enjoying his leisure. It is also employed by the Indians of South America, the Jibáros and others, during the performance of certain religious ceremonies. These Indians, according to the reports of Karsten, also smoke for pleasure, but use only imported tobacco, whereas that cultivated by themselves is reserved for religious purposes in order to accentuate the magic powers of the body, to increase its resistance against evil spirits, and as a narcotic for the production of dreams.

Its Modes of Employment
Snuff

The different modes of utilizing tobacco have not changed since Europeans began to know of the drug. This is especially the case with regard to the snuffing and smoking of tobacco, two methods of application which for a long time developed on parallel lines. In the year 1558, when tobacco was introduced into Portugal, the powdered leaf was stuffed into the nose. then, after Jean Nicot, the French ambassador at the Portuguese Court in 1560, had sent some seeds of the plant which he had cultivated himself to Catherine de' Medici in France, snuffing was the first mode of application and Herba Nicotiana was cultivated for the first time in the latter country. The Queen became patroness of the plant, which was at that time called Herba Medicea or Herba Catherinea. The poet and historian Buchanan directed a bitter epigram against this appelation. He said that this name would cause tobacco to lose all its good properties and transform them into poison, for Catherine was the scum, the pestilence, and the Medea of her century:

At Medice Catharina καθαρμα luesque suorum
Medea seculi sui
Ambitione ardens, Medicaeae nomine plantam
Nicotianam adulterat.

This queen also caused her sons, Francois II and Charles IX, when ill, to apply tobacco snuff as a medicinal remedy for headaches.[20] The "Tabac à priser," the "Panacée Cathérinaire" naturally became very popular at the Court of the Queen, both among the rich and very soon also among the people, and was employed against all kinds or real or imaginary diseases as well as to excite the nerves. At first it was a mere fashion, but afterwards became a fixed habit. At a later date Spanish sailors and soldiers spread the use of tobacco over other parts of the world. In the sixteenth century the Spanish priests had grown so accustomed to smoking and snuff-taking that they did not even refrain from indulging in this habit during Mass or when celebrating Communion. The dean and chapter of Seville therefore approached Pope Urban VIII, who in order to inhibit this scandalous abuse excommunicated those who smoked or snuffed tobacco (Espagnol, Spaniol) in the churches of Spain. This was the same Pope who in his leisure hours made bouquets and presented them to ladies of Rome. In 1650 Pope Innocent X issued an equally menacing edict against snuff-taking in the church of St. Peter in Rome, which was soiled thereby. In spite of all this, snuff-taking was continued to the verge of a mania.

The snuff-box, the tabatière, was an integral part of the costume of gentlemen from the seventeenth to the nineteenth century. It became an object of luxury. Made of porcelain, silver or gold, and decorated with precious stones, art gave it various forms which were in great demand. The English statesman Petersham had a different snuff-box for every day of the year, and was very angry if his valet did not give him the right one for the day in question. In the English Budget of 1822 the sum of £22,500 sterling is mentioned among the State expenses, this amount being spent by the British monarch on snuff-boxes which were dedicated to the noses of foreign ambassadors. Frederick II transformed his waistcoat pockets into snuff-boxes, and Napoleon, who was a very ardent snuff-taker, scattered large quantities of tobacco on his clothes. When during a sitting of his council he became nervous and found the regard of a high dignitary resting on him, he stretched out his arm and made a sign with his thumb and forefinger. The person in question then hurried to hand him his tabatière. The emporer played with it, scattered its contents over the table, and at last thoughtlessly placed it in his pocket. Occasionally several disappeared into his pocket in this manner. After the termination of the meeting, the Emperor, or Josephine, found them and sent them back to their owners. Frequently, however, they were exchanged, so that, for instance, instead of a wooden snuff-box, one made of gold studded with diamonds was returned. In order perhaps to avoid the loss of a souvenir the counsellors used snuff-boxes of cardboard or other material of little value.

In the course of the last century snuff-taking has lost many followers in Europe, but in other parts of the world the habit is still indulged in, for instance in the Caucasus by the Chewsuri women, in Turkey (Burmotu tobacco, Burmut), by the Afghans, Mongols, Tibetans, in Chinese Turkestan—every Shantu has his small gourd with tobacco hanging from his waist-band from which he takes a pinch from time to time—and ardently by the inhabitants of East Greenland and to a considerable extent by the women of the west coast.

In Africa this mode of application of tobacco is in vogue in many parts. The following will serve to prove this statement: In Nubia and Abyssinia the Somali and Danakils take snuff, frequently adding alkaline charcoal or an alkaline sodium salt (Soda, Atron, Magadi) to their tobacco. The latter tribe are also stated to add saltpetre to the snuff. The Oromó have small pouches for snuff (*nuschûk*) which is a mixture of tobacco and ashes. This particular custom exists also in Angola. It is especially remarkable because in this mode of utilizing tobacco, as in that of coca and betel, the people's instinct discovered the right way of augmenting the action of the drug, namely the use of an alkaline substance which sets free the active principle, in this case nicotine. Many African tribes smoke, take snuff, and also chew tobacco, for instance, the Wafiome, Wambugwe, and Warundi. The last-named, after having taken snuff, generally pinch their noses in the gap of a half-split piece of wood in order to prolong the effects. The Washashi and other peoples near the Victoria Nyanza, the Wakuafi, Wangori, Wataturi, Wapokomo, the Turkana of Lake Rudolf, the Nilotic tribes, all make use of tobacco. The negroes of the Congo and the Cameroons add to their imported Kentucky tobacco a third part of the alkaline ash of the shell of a pisang which has been roasted and reduced to a fine powder. The Munchis in the territory of the Agara smoke out of large clay pipes which pass from hand to hand during a meeting. Detzner observed others incessantly pouring the finely powdered tobacco out of leather pouches on the palms of their hands in order to stimulate their imagination by the sight of large doses. In the highlands of Angola tobacco is mainly smoked by the women. The men pass the pipe from mouth to mouth after having taken a few whiffs. They also take snuff in the form of finely powdered "ball-tobacco." The latter is prepared by pressing the fresh leaves between the hands and forming them into balls, which are then dried. This tobacco has a very marked exciting action. The Vey in Liberia, the Barotse, etc., also use tobacco, and in Morocco tobacco for snuffing is in great demand.

The Inglete Indians on the banks of the Yukon (Alaska) smoke tobacco, and also inhale it powdered from a box in their noses with the aid of a wooden pipe.

The Bonis in Guiana practice the peculiar custom of inhaling a concentrated extract of tobacco through the nose. The Uitotos on the banks of the Yapurá blow powdered tobacco into their own noses, or those of others, with the aid of tubes made of bone in the form of a cross. The tobacco is in the cavity of the tube and the end of the tube held by one in his mouth leads into the nose of the other.

The Jibáros and many other tribes of Ecuador smoke tobacco on festive occasions, and also take it through the nose in the form of an infusion or an extract prepared with saliva. The women imbibe it. Such tobacco fluids are employed not only on special occasions but also on ordinary days. The Jibáro washes his mouth very early in the morning with an infusion of ilex; he then boils some tobacco leaves, pours the decoction into the hollow of his hand, and repeatedly sucks the liquid up through the nose and lets it run off again through the mouth. By these means the head is said to be kept clear, the organism influenced favourably, and headaches and catarrhs avoided.

Chewing

There are various forms and modes of application of chewing-tobacco. English sailors in the middle of the seventeenth century were much addicted to its use. Admiral Monk, later Duke of Albemarle, who restored the English royal house, was a passionate tobacco-chewer. This form of the application of tobacco still obtains to some extent at the present day, but only in some classes of the population.

When tobacco is chewed or snuffed the active principles are extracted by the mucous membranes, in the one case of the nose and in the other of the mouth. The extracted nicotine-containing juice is absorbed in the nose and passes thence into the lymph canals. When tobacco is chewed the extract swallowed is absorbed by the mucous membranes of the stomach. In Europe waste tobacco useless for smoking is employed for the preparation of snuff and chewing-tobacco. Other waste substances are also added to snuff and the whole product is frequently impregnated with a tobacco-juice which is not always harmless. In other parts of the world chewing-tobacco is prepared in a far more simple manner. The Hova in Madagascar introduces powdered tobacco with an adroit movement of his hand between his lower lip and his teeth and chews it in this manner. The inhabitants of the interior use sauced leaves, i.e. leaves which have been soaked in tobacco juice, for the same purpose. The Somali chew or eat tobacco-leaves or small balls of tobacco and ashes. The North-Western Galla leave the tobacco-leaves to ferment, boil them, remove the juice by pressure and form the substance into bread-like lumps weighing 45 to 90 grammes. Occasionally cowdung is added. In Harar and South Arabia the women also chew tobacco. The Vey, the Golah, and the Pessy in Liberia triturate the tobacco with soap and the ashes of banana skins in small mortars. The mixture is preserved in sheep or goat horns with closed lids, an instinctively judicious precaution to prevent the evapouration of the nicotine. A small spoonful of this mixture is then cautiously inserted under the tongue.

The chewing of tobacco is also to be found in other parts of Africa, for instance in Tripoli, in the interior of Togo, etc. The same is also the case in Eastern Asia, for instance in the Malay Archipelago,

by the Dyaks, the Alfuru, who also smoke, in the Malay Peninsula,
etc. South American tribes also indulge in the chewing of tobacco.
Koch-Grünberg, for example, states that a Waíka kept a thick roll of
tobacco between his lower lip and his teeth and chewed it so thoroughly that the brown juice flowed down from both corners of this
mouth. After some time he removed the roll of tobacco and pushed it
into the mouth of a friend sitting next to him.

Chimó is a paste made of tobacco-juice which is inspissated by
boiling to the consistency of tar and to which ashes or soda, or occasionally opium, is added. This preparation is taken in doses of the size
of a pea by the men and women of Venezuela, the provinces of
Maracaibo, Trujillo, etc. The people state that it banishes hunger,
stimulates and soothes the spirits, and gives solace in all cases of physical and mental distress. A very considerable adaptation of the organism must have taken place to permit the absorption of this powerful
nicotine preparation which is taken frequently and in relatively strong
doses. In the course of an experiment where a person retained a dose
of the substance for ten minutes in his mouth a heaviness in the head
was experienced and the weakness of the legs became so marked that
he was hardly able to walk. The Arekunas in British Guiana prepare
chewing-tobacco from fresh leaves which are cut into small pieces
and black earth which is rich in saltpetre, and the Greenlanders mix
their tobacco with the remnants in their pipes for the same purpose.

There are two other variants of the habit, which consist of licking
and drinking tobacco.

The Uitotos and Miranyas, who inhabit the territory between the
Caqueta and the Putumayo, boil tobacco-leaves with water to a mass
of syrupy consistency which, when wrapped in leaves, can be preserved and sent away. In the evening the men meet and sit together
chewing coca. If an important matter has to be attended to, such as an
expedition for war or hunting, everyone dips his fore- and middle fingers into the pot of tobacco syrup and licks it from them. This licking
of tobacco corresponds to an oath.

The Jibáros drink tobacco-water, or an extract prepared with saliva, as a dream-producing narcotic. They retire into the forests in
order to enter into communication with their ancestors in the Rancho
specially reserved for this purpose. They remain there up to eight days
and return in an emaciated and fatigued state, for they eat nothing

save a roasted banana daily, but they are happy and content if the dreams are favourable. The medicine men of the Taulipáng and other South American tribes evoke in themselves a hallucinatory and visionary intoxication by the excessive smoking of strong tobacco and especially by drinking strong tobacco-juice. In this state the soul is separated from the body, according to the belief of the Indians, and after the return to normal conscoiusness the impression remains that what has been experienced is real.

Smoking

Many pages might be covered in this way with descriptions of the different means which various peoples of the earth employ when making use of tobacco. It would also be ascertained that without knowledge of the chemistry of tobacco man has invented all kinds of preventive measures, frequently effective, against the absorption of the combustion products of the smoke. In order to prevent them from reaching the mouth, for instance, he has made the smoke pass through a layer of water, or more primitively, as has been observed in Makaraká, the smoker placed a small wisp of finely divided fibres into his mouth through which he inhaled the smoke. Tribes in the territory of the White Nile suck the smoke through spherical or pear-like gourds which are full of the fibres of *hibiscus*, which is similar to hemp.

Along the south-east coast of New Guinea from the Torres Straits to the East Cape the inhabitants smoke at social meetings with the aid of the "Baubau", a tube $1^1/_2$ metres long which is open at one end and has a small aperture at the other. A bag or cone made of the leaf of a tree and filled with tobacco is ignited and inserted into the small opening. The chief smoker sucks the tube full of smoke, which his neighbours one after the other inhale in their turn until no smoke is left in the tube. The chief smoker sets to work again until all present, children included, are satisfied.

The natives of the Bismarck Archipelago, for instance in New Pomerania, prepare their own large cigars. They hold them in their fists, and after having blown through them several times, inhale the smoke into the lungs.

The Maoris of New Zealand, both men and women, smoke, and if the child which is carried by its mother on her back cries too loudly, the pipe is pushed into its mouth.

In Liberia women and children open the mouth as wide as possible so that tobacco smoke may be blown into it.

At the "festival of the men" of the Jibáros, on the banks of the Rio Pasteza, the youth who is about to become an adult is prepared for the ceremony by fasting. Cigar-smoke is then blown into his mouth with the aid of a tube by the master of ceremonies. The fumes of a whole cigar are thus swallowed by the novice and pass into his stomach. This process is repeated from six to eight times on both days of the festival and exercises a very powerful influence on the young man, the more so because tobacco juice is also served. Narcosis sets in, and in this state he sees spirits which prophesy his future and endow him with strength, knowledge, and happiness. In some tribes the master of ceremonies places the burning end of the cigar in his mouth and the other in the mouth of the novice, and blows the smoke, which is then swallowed by the latter.

The inhabitants of the islands of the Torres Straits, those of the western part of New Guinea, and the Sakai already smoked leaves similar to tobacco before becoming acquainted with Europeans. A plant similar to tobacco was smoked by the Tlinkit before they were discovered, and Lieutenant Whidbey, of Vancouver, observed tobacco plantations in the Chatham Straits. It is very probable that the leaves of *nicotiana suaveolens* were smoked in New Holland before Europeans arrived there.

The "normal" manner of smoking a pipe, a cigar, or a cigarette also offers many variations, from the typical ejection of the smoke from the mouth to the ingenious methods which modern cigarette smokers, adult and juvenile, have invented. One emits the inhaled smoke after some time from his nose, another, the "lung-smoker," inhales it, like the Indian of the Rocky Mountains, far into the respiratory organs and gives it off in the form of a large cloud, a third swallows the smoke and ejects it unexpectedly at an opportune moment. These artists in smoking do not dream that very frequently these pretty tricks have harmful results to which they may one day fall victims.

Women and children also participate in smoking to a great extent, not only as in former times those of primitive and distant countries, but also those living in civilized environments. The older women of Bogotá in Columbia are not satisfied with smoking cigarettes like ladies of the social standing, but also take cigars, and in order to increase the pleasure frequently insert the burning end into their mouths. In Paraguay mothers insert the cigar into the mouth of their infants, and the children of the Buryats at the southern end of the Lake Baikal, even when hardly able to stand on their feet, smoke tobacco mixed with the bark of trees. The men, women and children of the Manguns on the banks of the lower Amur, of the Ostyaks, Samoyeds, and other tribes of north-eastern Asia, are passionately addicted to smoking. The smoke of an abominable tobacco, Machorka, is swallowed by the Ostyaks and then ejected again. The same is found in the Indian Islands, for instance the Nicobars, Philippines, Solomons, etc., where the children already smoke shortly after having been weaned. This is also the case with the Australian aborigines.

This craving for tobacco which the women of countries far from civilization in Asia, Melanesia, Polynesia, Africa, and America exhibit and satisfy—only a few tribes forbid the habit to women—has invaded the female sex in countries where the modern spirit, the spirit of to-day, the spirit of emancipation from ancient prejudices reigns. It is not a question of some old peasant woman inserting an old and dirty pipe inherited from her deceased husband into her toothless mouth, but of the mainly juvenile female flower of the nation, the *"Emancipata fumans vulgaris,"* who should bear fruit in time to come, but frequently fails to do so because the foolish consumption of cigarettes has impregnated the sexual organs with smoke and nicotine and keeps them in a state of irritation and inflammation. Such women as homely vestals should nourish a fire of quite another sort, for their mouth is ordained for other things than to be transformed into a smoking chimney and to smell of tobacco juice.

The Conquest of Mankind by Tobacco

After the introduction of tobacco into Europe and the spread of the knowledge of its properties the increasing demand for the drug was soon in greater part met by European cultivation of the plant. The quantities imported into Europe by Portuguese, Spanish, French, and English sailors in the middle of the sixteenth century were but small. At the time when Walter Raleigh in 1586 brought tobacco from Virginia to England there were in Portugal whole plantations, the seeds probably having been obtained from Yucatan. Tobacco was also grown in some parts of Germany, in Suhl even in 1559; but it was not before

the time of the Thirty Years' War that its cultivation was of any importance. At the beginning it was only used for horticultural or purely
medicinal purposes, but it soon became a factor of economic importance on account of the increasing consumption of tobacco as a stimulant. Only two of the forty-one species of Nicotiana, *nicotiana tabacum*
and *nicotiana rustica*, are cultivated for this purpose at the present day.
In all temperate and subtropical climates there are plantations of these
two species and the consumption of them is enormous. Statistics, however, can only be given for civilized countries. It is impossible to estimate the amounts consumed by the producers from the depths of the
virgin forest to the unknown tobacco-fields of distant lands.

The following countries consume between 2 to 3 kg. annually per
head of population on a decreasing scale: Holland, the United States,
Belgium, Switzerland, Austria-Hungary, less than 2 kg. in Germany,
Australia, Scandinavia, Russia, France, Italy, Spain, etc.

Many obstacles were met with before the plantations necessary to
meet the increasing demand could be started and before tobacco was
able to conclude its conquest of the world. Very early the always un-
wise restrictions of Governments became manifest which frequently
made use of barbaric methods at a time before tobacco was recognized
as a substance of high economic and financial value for collecting
taxes.

In all ages all artificial desires have from time to time been opposed by the severity of the law. The use of tobacco also had mighty
enemies animated by reasons of sentiment, political economy, and
religious scruples, but they nevertheless failed in their aim of preventing the consumption of tobacco. I have already described the manner
in which the Pope proceeded by interdictions and punishments against
tobacco-users in the churches of Spain and Rome. It was of no avail,
for in 1725 the Pope had to capitulate to the weed. Benedict XIII,
who himself liked to take snuff, annulled all edicts which had hitherto been issued against the "dry drunkenness," as it was called in
Germany, in order to avoid the scandalous spectacle of dignitaries of
the Church hastening out in order to take a few clandestine whiffs in
some corner away from spying eyes.

In Germany also there were many prohibitions. In Lüneburg in
1691 the death penalty was still in force against smoking, "the abominable habit of drinking tobacco." In Saxony it was forbidden to smoke

in the street and in stage-coaches, and by an edict of 1723 in Berlin also. In the eighteenth century an edict was issued in Saxe-Gotha in terms of paternal solicitude as follows: "In view of the fact that many persons make use of tobacco in an inopportune and exaggerated manner, which is very harmful, parents should prohibit its use in their families to prevent them from coming to harm. A person excessively addicted to this evil should be reprimanded like any other drunkard or handed over to the authorities for severe punishment. Likewise tobacco must not be sold on credit or be the object of debts, and those who sell it on credit will be severely punished."

In Transylvania and Hungary in 1689, a fine of 300 florins was imposed for the offence of smoking, and in the former country the cultivation of tobacco was punished by the confiscation of the fortune of the offender. In Switzerland, especially in Berne, the smoking of tobacco was regarded as a grave criminal offence in 1660, and in 1849 a law was promulgated in Canton Valais which punished smoking by youths under twenty years of age with a fine or in case of repetition of the offence with imprisonment. Towards the end of the nineteenth century this legislation was formally renewed, with the result that the lower official of the State pointed out its uselessness on account of the popularity of tobacco. In Holland the passion for smoking had increased to such an extent that the students indulged in it to excess, in spite of the abjurations of the faculty of medicine, which condemned tobacco because it "blackened the brain." This is a fine example of the many stupid but amusing professorial dicta, about which a book might well be written. The students while away their time in "tobacco houses." At that period children might be seen at table with pipes in their mouths. In England in 1603 James I wrote his "Misocapnus" (the tobacco-hater), in which he attributes all evils to tobacco. Very soon, however, he imposed a tax on tobacco, as did Charles I, and proved in this way that he was a good financier. In 1652 the cultivation of tobacco in England was prohibited for the benefit of the American colonies. In Sweden smoking was prohibited by Gustav III, the king who confessed that he hated nothing on earth more than tobacco and the German language!

In Turkey tobacco first became known in 1605, and in 1642 it was taken as snuff. The clergy protested because it violated the laws of the Koran. The nose of the tobacco-user was pierced, the stem of a pipe passed through the hole, and he was ridden through the street on a donkey. Murad (Amurath) IV in 1620 punished the smoking of tobacco with the death-penalty, to be immediately carried out in one of the ancient forms agreeable to God. Mohammed IV permitted it once more. In Persia the smoking of tobacco was in old times punished by death, and in Russia the Tzar Michael Fedorovitch had done to death everyone of his beloved subjects on whom tobacco was found, or who dealt in it or drank, i.e. smoked it. Their possessions were sold and the amount realized forfeited to the Imperial Treasury. Castigation was sometimes applied, and also the ingenious method of cutting off the nose, which was practised in Persia and Abyssinia. The Tzar Alexei Mikhailovitch had everyone on whom tobacco was found tortured until he disclosed the source from which he had obtained it.

The Mexican State of Tabasco quite recently put an Act into force by which everyone who smoked in public was liable to a special tax. Public smoking is placed on a level with public drunkenness.

There must have been some reason for these rigorous prohibitions, which were not merely of a political or private nature. For in the case of tobacco the State taxed the drug in its own interest far earlier and to a greater degree than in that of any other substance of the same kind. On the other hand, the smoker spends less on the consumption of tobacco than, for instance, on alcoholic beverages, or other private amusements. State duties on tobacco were imposed at a very early date. James I, the tobaccophobe, already levied a tax of 6s. 10d. on every hundredweight, and in France, where smoking became popular in the reign of Louis XIII, the pound was taxed 30 sous. Following the example of England, where in the reign of Charles I, in order to restore the finances, the colonial planters were forced to sell tobacco to the Government at a fixed price, other countries also imposed heavy duties, for instance Portugal in 1664, Austria in 1670, France in 1674, etc. When in Russia death-penalties and mutilations proved of no avail the Tzar Peter the Great sold to England a licence to import tobacco into Russia for £15,000 sterling.

Humboldt states that in the province of Cumana in Venezuela the cultivation of tobacco was, after the imposition of State control in 1779, mainly confined to a small district. In Mexico this was also the case in Orizaba and Cordova. The whole crop had to be sold to the State. It was for this reason that in order to avoid fraudulent trading, the plantations were limited to one territory. Surveyors scoured the country and destroyed every plantation outside the prescribed limits. They also brought an action against every poor Indian who took the risk of smoking a cigar the tobacco of which he had grown in his own garden and which had not passed through the hands of the Government.

Taxes on tobacco have continued until the present day to be an important source of revenue for many countries. At the beginning of this century France derived from its tobacco monopoly a clear profit of over 323 million francs, and the import duty on the raw and finished product in other countries without a monopoly reaches very large sums.

Its Good and Evil Effects

Now that we have described the motives which have created friends and enemies of tobacco and abstainers from its use during the course of the centuries, it only remains for us to consider the medical reasons for and against smoking. Why does man smoke, chew, and snuff tobacco? The description of de las Casas, previously quoted, of the habituation of the Spaniards to the smoking habit which they saw practised by the Indians and could not refrain from imitating, closes with the following words: "I do not know what benefit they derive from it." Others answer this question at a later date. Molière makes Sganarelle say of snuff in the *Festin de Pierre:* "It not only refreshes and cleanses the brain, but also leads the soul to virtue and teaches honesty. Tobacco calls forth the desire for honour and virtue in all who make use of it. Aristotle and all philosophers may say what they like, there is nothing like tobacco. It is the habit of the best people, and those who live without tobacco are not worth keeping alive." Such intemperate language may be excused in the case of a layman, especially as it may be partly ironical, but the Dutch physician, Bontekoe, who lived at about the same time as Molière, used similar words of praise: "Nothing is more necessary and beneficial to life and health than the smoke of tobacco. It gladdens the heart in solitude and relieves a sedentary life of all discomforts." The plant is described by others as an ornament to the earth, a present from Olympus, deserving for good reasons the praise of all the world.

Planta beata! decus terrarum, munus Olympi,
. . . vix sanior herba
Extitit et meritos jam nunc gratantur honores
Africa gens, Asiaque ingens, Europaeaque nostra.

Many pages might be covered with verses alone, the product of the enthusiasm of snuff-taking or smoking poets of the last two centuries. But others poured many drops of gall into this sparkling wine. Molière on account of his eulogy of tobacco was violently abused by Cohausen in the now famous book, *Satyrical Thoughts of the Pica nasi or the Longings of the Concupiscent Nose, i.e. the Abuse and the Injurious Effects of Taking Snuff,* in which Molière is called a clown and rouge. "Tobacco is a great God in Brazil, and was cultivated and born in Virginia. He is a king in the vegetable realm and is sovereign of all parts of the world. All over the world the smoking lips of all nations sing his praises, thousands of hands are occupied in making pipes and snuff-boxes for his service; and not less numerous noses, his slaves, pay tribute in the face of the whole world. He is a hero who extends his power over the male sex and has in a hitherto unknown manner established an influence among women. I do not know whether he is the father or the stepfather of health. He is clandestinely allied with disease or triumphs over it. He is a true companion both of idleness and business, a courtier of princes and a comrade of the peasants in the sheepfold, a helper of the armies in the field and of the muses in the study." The author becomes very angry indeed when speaking of the snuff-taking peasants: "Even fellows behind the plough cannot abstain from inhaling the cherished plant with their flat noses. They love to scratch and besmirch their hairy nostrils with this stuff, and noses which hitherto were used only to the odour of cart-grease now smell 'Spanish.'" The evil effects of snuff-taking are described: "The sense of smell has in many cases been weakened by the abuse of snuff, and very frequently lost altogether. This evil habit has caused the loss of eyesight, and many have become deaf. It is especially injurious to the brain as well as to the chest, the windpipe and the lungs."

In 1627 the French historian Sorel briefly and concisely calls tobacco the dessert of the devil. At an early date tobacco was accused of being a disturber of the health of the people in England, and in 1585 the historian Camden wrote: "At that time [i.e. in the reign of Queen

Elizabeth] the people began to smoke out of pipes very frequently, and expended therein large sums of money; so that the impression was soon gained that the bodies of the English had degenerated to the state of barbarians."

Extremely numerous complaints have been put forward from those times to the present day with respect to the injurious effects of tobacco. These effects must be studied from a critical and a clinical point of view.

The activity of no other substance described in this book is subjected in such a degree as that of tobacco to modifying influences, the result of the varying composition of the product and its transformation during application. It may indeed be stated that the series of substances from opium to the stimulating purines must as a whole be regarded as nearly constant in their composition and their greater or lesser activity remains within narrow limits. On the other hand the active content in tobacco varies very much and the effects of these variations do not fail to become apparent even when individual resistance is left out of consideration. Moreover, tobacco as soon as it is being smoked ceases to be tobacco in the botanical and chemical sense of the word. It emits with a part of the active substances originally present a number of gaseous products which also play an important part. It will readily be understood that the production of these extremely various substances varies with the individual manner of smoking, and that they are all apt to be introduced into the organism and to give rise to more or less acute toxic symptoms, or gradually call forth effects differing in strength and form. We need only consider the differing aspects of some of the usual forms of tobacco-smoking. There is the short pipe, the pipe with a long stem and a cleansing tube, the very long student's pipe, the oriental water-pipe which absorbs the products of condensation of the smoke, the cigar, and the cigarette. Without any detailed chemical explanation it will easily be understood that the final biological consequences are influenced by these different circumstances under which the smoke is produced. The following substances are in this manner apt to affect the human organism: nicotine, nicoteine, nicotimine, nicotelline, the recently discovered nicotoine, and isonicotoine, a nitrogen-free acid oil with isovalerianic acid, products of the salt or aromatic caustic of the tobacco with unknown content, pyridin bases, prussic acid, and carbon monoxide. Even this list does not exhaust the number of substances produced by the combustion of tobacco. The extremely various forms of nicotinism are influenced by all kinds of conditional and determining factors. Apart from individual susceptibility, the manner of smoking is the most important of these. It is the latter which causes the mucous membranes of the respiratory organs to absorb more or less of the active substances.

In my own view cigarette-smoking is the most dangerous manner of utilizing tobacco.

The decisive factor in the effects of tobacco, desired or undesired, is nicotine, which is contained to the extent of from 2 to over 7 per cent, according to the kind of tobacco, and it matters little whether it passes directly into the organism or whether it is smoked. Four to five milligrammes of this alkaloid are contained and become active in the average cigarette or cigar. The "smoke-swallowers," for instance, the Koryaks of Eastern Asia, the Yakuts, the Motus of New Guinea, or the Papuans from Milne Bay to Teste Island with their *kira,* and others, exhibit acute symptoms of intoxication such as perspiration, dyspnœa, coughing, etc., on account of the large amount of smoke ingested. Among the Chukches total intoxication with collapse, etc., has been observed after deglutition of 6–7 whiffs of tobacco. Whymper saw the same occur among the Malemutts near Norton Sound in Alaska, and we have all seen this for ourselves in certain smokers.

The carbon monoxide contained in smoke probably plays an important part in the production of these effects, for 1 gr. of cigar or pipe tobacco furnishes more than 70 cc. of this gas. The noxious action is augmented if in addition to tobacco other substances are smoked which are liable to give off carbon monoxide, such as hair (among the Samoyeds), wooden scrapings and aspen-bark (among the Yakuts), straw and wood (Burma), willow bark (Malemutts), or if, as in Angola and Liberia when tobacco is lacking, charcoal alone is smoked. The Bari in the Equatorial Province, the A-Sendé, and the Nuer smoke tobacco and charcoal in the same manner. In South America the tobacco is formed into cigars with the aid of fibres, e.g. of *curatari guayensis* or *lecitys ollaria.* There are many other specialties in the chemical constitution of tobacco or its smoke which are apt to render its use disagreeable, whether at once or after a lapse of time.

Abstracting from cases where tobacco is smoked to excess or in an injurious manner, a series of agreeable effects remain which have more or less consciously attracted mankind to its use. It must be pointed out that the attraction of tobacco is not exercised with that vigour and inexorable constraint which we have remarked in the case of the narcotic substances described in this work. If the use of tobacco has to be stopped for medical or other reasons, no suffering of the body or morbid desire for the drug appears. The consumption of tobacco is an enjoyment which man is free to renounce, and when he indulges in it he experiences its benevolent effects on his spiritual life.

Smoking does not call forth an exultation of internal well-being as does the use of wine, but it adjusts the working condition of the mind and the disposition of many mentally active persons to a kind of serenity or "quietism" during which the activity of thought is in no way disturbed, and from a physical point of view a certain calmness of movement occurs. In his letters written during his travels in Turkey, Moltke remarked that the tobacco-pipe was the magic wand which changed the Turk from one of the most turbulent of men into a lover of peace. Although the action of tobacco in most cases consists in banishing vacancy of mind and boredom, so that the layman has the impression of a slight narcosis, it is nevertheless a mild excitation. The latter dominates or substitutes other normal or natural states of excitation of the cerebral centres and directs them into other channels so that the final impression is one of self-forgetfulness without any irritation of the brain.

The smoking of cigarettes is somewhat different in its action and employment from that of the pipe or the cigar, which is the modern symbol of confidence and intimacy. The smoking of cigarettes is very extensively practised at present. It was during the Crimean war that French and English officers learnt this convenient mode of smoking from their Turkish allies. The fashion soon spread over the whole world, and is practised especially by the young to such a degree that the results of this excess have given rise to anxiety in medical circles. In England an Act was recently passed which prohibits smoking by persons under the age of sixteen, orders the guardians of the law to prosecute offenders, and forbids the sale of tobacco and cigarettes to persons under this age. In Norway a similar law has been put into force, and the State of Arkansas has taken more severe measures still. These are actuated by the best intentions, but unfortunately are without success.

As George Forster pointed out more than a hundred years ago in his treatise on "sweet-stuffs," young people are generally inspired by vanity to appear like grown-ups, and to this end make use of these substances. The youthful imitator experiences none of these sensations which appeal to the adult smoker. His mental activity, limited in depth and breadth, does not need a chemical impulse to put its total output at his disposal. It is not possible for irritants or stimulants to call forth more than is actually there; they cannot give rise to something which can only be the product of a further natural development. If in spite of this an artificial irritant of this kind habitually exercises its influence for some time it will, even in the case of a good constitution, result in material modifications not only of the brain but also of the organic functions dominated thereby if the use of the drug is not stopped in time. Only interesting lessons on human physiology in the schools will avail against the cigarette-mania among juveniles. This kind of instruction is certain to be very beneficial to the race, far more than the development of "physical culture" which is so much in vogue at the present day.

There is no hope for the inveterate cigarette-smoker. Not even the prospect of premature death serves to bring about a lessening of the passion, even if the organism has given warning in this respect. I have frequently made this observation in many cases where I have been consulted. *Volenti non fit injuria!* Such foolish folk, who would rather die of nicotinism than curb their passion for smoking, are also subject to predestination. Their ashes supply them with the final object of their desires.

Physical Disturbances Due to Tobacco

Even though less than 70 per cent of the nicotine were to pass into the smoke, this amount together with the other substances rich in energy which pass into the lymph-canals represents a sum of active principles whose absorption by the organism cannot be ignored if smoking is indulged in to excess. The innate regulating forces concealed in the organism of which man is unaware, and which are a part of his total vital energy, are always ready to compensate or repair disorders due to internal or external injuries. But if these latter are incessantly repeated the compensating force has to be at work at all times in the organism. Naturally traces of this overwork are apt to occur, similar to functional callosities or scars, but the organs in question are able for a long time to preserve the external appearance of physiological and functional health.

As I have stated in the preceding pages, it has been sought to explain these inexplicable processes by another obscure expression, that of "habituation," which many experiences of daily life have made a current term. In the same way the fact that in some cases the compensation of the initial effects due to an injurious factor does not occur by the words "idiosyncrasy," "increased insensibility," and "intolerance." The action of nicotine especially, more than that of all the other substances previously studied, gives rise to two series of contradictory phenomena. Animals subjected to the repeated action of nicotine exhibit a state of habituation to the poison after a greater or lesser lapse of time. This habituation to the drug takes place very slowly in the case of young animals, which on the whole tolerate the substance to a lesser degree. There are also, however, series of experiments where habituation was completely lacking. After 10 to 100 injections of nicotine the reactions were the same as after the initial doses, both in nature and intensity. In animal cases of immunity towards certain modifications of a material order can also be ascertained, as for instance lesions of the aorta.

It is a well-known fact that the toleration of nicotine may reach a very great degree, although its intoxicating power is fifteen times as great as that of coniine, the active principle of hemlock. It is therefore not necessary to cite particular examples. It is also well known that inveterate smokers are not exempt from the symptoms of acute intoxication if they overpass the limit of toleration. It is, moreover, common knowledge that the use of tobacco for smoking and chewing does not necessitate a progressive increase of the dose as in the case in other toxic substances and that the symptoms due to withdrawal of tobacco, if they occur at all, are easily overcome. These latter consist of an extreme feeling of discomfort and eventually bad humour and dejection. It is very exceptionally that graver symptoms occur. There are very many experiences of everyday life which apprise us of the intoleration of tobacco, especially by juveniles. It is stated that the Arabs are not able to smoke our tobacco at all, because a few whiffs give rise to vertigo and headaches. Nervous people and those suffering from heart and vascular diseases and digestive troubles also exhibit a diminished resistance to tobacco.

The consequences of the abuse of tobacco are more numerous and various than in the case of any similar substance. There is no organ whose function may not suffer, and no functional disorder whose origin is not recognized as a manifestation of nicotinism. The statements of ignorant persons that a very advanced age can be reached in spite of smoking are true, but it is just as true that old age is not reached as a result of excessive smoking. And if when regarding the toxicosis of tobacco not death but disease only is taken into consideration, every attempt to acquit tobacco fails before the inexorable facts to the contrary. For there are hardly any chapters of pathology which are not connected in some way with the abuse of tobacco. Observations have been made of the inhibition of physical and intellectual development in the case of 187 students who smoked. It seems to me that, even if the importance attached to these investigations were not decisive, the whole manner of the action of tobacco-smoke and the substances contained therein is liable to be effective in this way, for instance with respect to the capacity of the lungs. It has repeatedly been observed that an increase of the excretion of sugar in the urine follows from smoking. It cannot be doubted at the present day that an alteration of a pathological kind in the walls of the vessels appears as a result of excessive consumption of tobacco, and this has also been proved in animals subjected to chronic nicotine poisoning. Aneurysmal dilatations, roughness, and calcareous incrustations on the large arteries have been ascertained. The muscular fibres of the middle artery are subjected to necrotic modifications, the cells of the muscles are replaced by calcareous deposits. The vessels become friable, and other parts of the arterial system, such as for instance the crural artery, also suffer from necrosis.

The heart is affected to a specially grave degree in both old and young, but particularly in persons between forty and fifty years of age who are passionate smokers. They suffer from intense palpitations which vary according to the degree of the intoxication from a harmless irregularity without consequences to cardiac delirium, the latter, however, being very rare. Tachycardia at the beginning occurs especially at night. Nevertheless Egyptian cigarettes are said to reduce the frequency of the pulse. Disagreeable and even painful sensations in the region of the heart, a sense of oppression in the chest, more rarely typical attacks of angina pectoris with loss of consciousness, the nicotinic origin of which has lately been contested, are also apt to set in. It must at present remain an open question whether anatomical alterations of the vagus nerve are present in these cases, as animal experiments seem to have proved. Gradually cardiac dilatation and hypertrophy are also liable to result. Total abstinence from tobacco frequently removes the cardiac symptoms. In some cases the acceleration of the pulse with irregularity remains.

Asthmatic disturbances and a modification of the respiratory type frequently in the form of sigh-like inspirations occurring at intervals are independent of the former symptoms. Spitting blood is rare. The visual disturbances which may set in are very numerous,[21] for instance inequality of the pupils, reduction of the central acuity of vision, colour-blindness in the middle of the field of vision, retrobulbar neuritis, and blindness. These symptoms disappear after several months if the use of tobacco is suppressed, but may leave traces, or, as was observed in the case of a chewer of tobacco, remain as total blindness. The latter also occurred in a man who smoked over 30 cigars a day.

The effects of tobacco on the nervous system are also extremely various. It is stated that non-smokers in higher schools make greater progress than those who smoke. Children up to fifteen years of age who smoked were less intelligent, lazier and exhibited an inclination for alcoholic beverages. Adult smokers to excess frequently suffer from a feeling of oppression in the head, vertigo, insomnia, aversion to work, abnormal temper, mental irritability, and also neuralgias in numerous branches of the nerves, troubles of motility such as muscular trembling, weakness of the sphincters, and cramps.

It has frequently been alleged that the chewing of tobacco in the form of roll tobacco or snuff in the northern parts of the world is the cause of mental diseases. In some parts amounts of 20–27 gr. per day are consumed. Disorders of this kind are stated to be rare in smokers of tobacco. These morbid mental states are said to begin with a premonitory state of about three months' duration, principally characterized by depression, anguish, and insomnia. Hallucinations, illusions, and suicidal intentions, at a later period alternative states of excitation and depression, follow. It is said that no cure is possible in serious cases after five to six months. Some time ago I already expressed my doubts as to the foundation of a precise description of nicotine psychosis[22] and I still maintain the same opinion. A medium exists between these two adverse opinions to the effect that tobacco is liable to give rise to mental diseases including epilepsy and neurasthenia in psychopathic persons.

Other symptoms of nicotinism have occasionally been mentioned, such as motor aphasia for several hours, and also amnesia. Auditory disorders are certainly caused thereby. It is with good reason that states of congestion of the middle ear tract with symptoms of tinnitus aurium and other local noises and deafness of both ears have been attributed to the abuse of tobacco.

It is certain also that occasionally a reduction and even the disappearance of sexual generative power takes place. Women who smoke frequently suffer from troubles of menstruation and other grave affections of the sexual apparatus. Granular pharyngeal disorders and inflammations frequently accompanied by leucoplacia, disorder of the digestive functions especially on account of swallowing the "tobacco-saliva," intestinal catarrhs, atrophic inflammations of the nose, and in the case of cigarette smokers who exhale through the nose, of the trachea also, and even diseases of the pancreas must be counted among the consequences of nicotine.

Substitutes for Tobacco

Many proposals have been made for withdrawing the venom from tobacco. The simplest idea of denicotinizing the leaves has been realized in quite a number of processes. Castrated tobacco has been prepared in this way, as with other similar substances. Some people smoke cigars without nicotine. If they find pleasure in doing so they are thought to be congratulated, although the impression persists that this is not the case. Moreover, toxic effects from nicotine-free tobacco have recently been described.

Other methods consist of breaking the habit by creating a loathing for tobacco-smoke, for instance by gargling with 0.25 per cent solution of silver nitrate. This was suggested by a probably not quite normal medical man, and the smoker after a short time is apt to suffer from a bluish-black complexion.

The peoples of those countries where tobacco cannot be obtained in sufficient quantities have adopted other measures and smoke different plants. I have already mentioned some of these. The people of Paraná and Rio Grande do Sul use the wood of *aristolochia triangularis* and *galeata,* and in parts of Brazil the dried leaves of *anthurium oxycarpum;* the Washamba employ the powdered leaves of *carica papaya* and the Hottentots those of *leonotis Leonurus*. In Mexico the stigmas and the wool of the common maize are smoked. In different parts of America the leaves and bark of the *vaccineum stamineum*, the bark of *salix purpurea, cornus stolonifera, arctostaphylos glauca, kalmia latifolia,* and *chimaphila umbellata* are used instead of tobacco. The Cholos Indians occasionally smoke the leaves and wood of a solanaceæ, *cestrum parqui (palguin)* which occurs in Chile and the south of Brazil, and in other parts of the country *caltha palustris, arbutus uva ursi, plygonum orientale,* and similar plants are utilized, not forgetting the cane which juveniles set alight and "smoke."

Several substances are also employed as substitutes for snuff, for instance the leaves of *anthurium oxycarpum* which when dried smell like vanilla, and other irritating powders, including the sneezing powder "Schneeberger Tobacco," which contains besides sweet marjoram, melilotus, and lavender, the root of hellebore. The Akkawai in Guiana chew the leaves of species of *lacis* which have been roasted over an open fire.

The natives of the Besoeki district of Java add the leaves and the stem of a certain ash-tree to their tobacco. It is stated that the smoke which is produced can in no way be distinguished from that of glowing opium. If this mixture is smoked an agreeable state is experienced as in opium-smoking, but the state of depression to which the latter gives rise is entirely absent. If this addiction to the tobacco really consists of the leaves of a species of ash-tree, then the effects stated above do not in the least agree with the results of previous experience of this plant.

The use of tobacco, which has made its way thanks to the spirit of imitation as well as to its peculiar effects, has vanquished humanity and will continue to reign until the end of the world.

Tobacco has surpassed the limits of a medical plant. It has penetrated far into the world and among mankind, escaping from the apothecaries, whence it had been banished, in spite of the penalties inflicted on its addicts.

"Defendons à toute personne de vendre du tabac sinon aux

apothicaires et par ordonnance de médecin à peine de quatre-vingts livres parisis d'amende."

These were the words of a police regulation of 1635. The cornucopia of the law has provided us also with an ordinance containing regulations for the sale of tobacco to juveniles. Paragraph 340 of the projected German penal code (1925) is as follows:

> Whosoever supplies tobacco containing nicotine to a person under the age of sixteen for his or her own use in the absence of a person in charge of his or her education or a representative of the latter shall be punished by a term of imprisonment not exceeding three months or a fine.

In my opinion smoking by juveniles, at least for the greater part of them, is most obnoxious to the organism. A paragraph of the penal code will not be able to inhibit the abuse of tobacco, especially if it be not adequately framed. The person who supplies the tobacco without authority is punished. But if it is the father or guardian who gives a cigarette to a fifteen-year-old boy, he is not liable to a penalty, although the deed and the aim of the punishment are the same. It seems to me that "the person in charge of education" should be liable to punishment for the reasons given above. And moreover, is the smoking of denicotinized tobacco absolutely harmless? This cannot be proved, as I have already pointed out.

Abstinence from tobacco as a result of a subjective point of view must be allowed for, like every other negative passion, such as hatred of women, abstinence from alcohol, etc. But this applies to the individual only. If the state of mankind must be improved, there are really more important tasks to accomplish, such as the improvement of conditions of work which are liable to shorten the lives of thousands of men. It is really immaterial to know whether the smoking of a cigar or cigarette did or did not give rise to agreeable sensations in the case of, let us say, Goethe, Tolstoy, or a motor-car manufacturer, but it is of the greatest importance to decide whether abstainers are justified in interdicting the temperate use of tobacco to others. No one, however, is in a position to penetrate into the complexity of the individual life of his neighbour with its all-important actions and reactions, and individual aversion to any agreeable sensation does not give a man the right to measure his neighbour's peck by his own bushel. Neither violence, mockery, nor contempt have been able to rob the reasonable consumption of tobacco of the halo with which it is surrounded. And it is worthy of general esteem if foolish men do not by abuse transform it into poison.

PARICA

The Ottomacs of the Upper Orinoco, the Guahibos, the Paravilhanos, the tribes of the lower Amazon, the Múras, Mauhés, and the Amaguas and the Ticunas on the banks of the upper reaches of the Amazon at times employ the powder of the *Paricá* (cohobba, niopo) in a manner similar to tobacco, as snuff. It is prepared from the seeds of a leguminous plant of the botanical order Mimoseae, not, as was formerly believed an *inga,* but, as is now certain, the *acacia niopo (piptadenia peregrina).* The seeds are dried in the sun, crushed in wooden mortars and preserved in bamboo tubes. The Paravilhanos and Ottomacs sometimes also subject the material to a process of fermentation before crushing. Humboldt states that the substance is also kneaded with manioc flour and burnt chalk prepared from shells and the whole mass dried over the fire. The resulting small cakes are powdered when required.

These tribes celebrate every year at harvest-time a festival lasting several days which has a partly religious character, and includes the consumption of enormous quantities of liquor. The Brazilians call this festival Quarantena. They imbibe large amounts of *caysûma* and *cashiri,* fermented beverages which give rise to heavy drunkenness, or cashasa, i.e. rum, if this is obtainable. After a short time they are in a state of semi-inebriety, and then begin to take Paricá snuff. With this end in view they assemble in pairs, everyone with a tube containing Paricá in his hand, and after having performed some incomprehensible and doubtless religious mummeries everyone blows the contents of his tube with all his strength into the nostrils of his partner.

The effects produced in these generally dull and silent people are extraordinary. They become very garrulous, and sing, scream, and jump about in wild excitement. After calming down they go on drinking again, and in this way a state of excitation alternates for days on end with one of depression.

The Mauhés and probably other tribes use Parciá medicinally as a prophylactic against fever which reigns during the intermediate months between the dry and rainy seasons. When a dose is to be applied a small amount of the hard substance is rubbed to a powder in a flat bowl and inhaled into the nostrils with the aid of the stalks of two vulture-feathers tied together with cotton. Other appliances in the form of a Y are also employed in order to inhale the substance into both nostrils simultaneously, thus giving rise to the effects described above.

I believe the effects of Paricá to consist mainly in a violent irritation of the mucous membrane of the nose, calling forth acute sensations of burning or pain therein. It must be regarded as improbable that there are active principles capable of affecting the brain in the genus of plants in question. There are, however, on the other hand leguminous plants which contain in their seeds or other parts saponins capable of irritating the tissues and destroying the cells, and for this reason may serve medicinally for the destruction of intestinal worms. The irritating action of the albumen which is peculiar to leguminous seeds cannot be taken into consideration, because this does not set in until after the lapse of several hours.

ARSENIC

Habituation to arsenic may take place to considerable degree. In the treatment of patients who need arsenic the possibility of this habituation not only makes possible the toleration of the large doses but finally renders them indispensable. In cases of psoriasis 10 gr. of arsenious acid may be taken during a certain time. This habituation also creates arsenic-eaters. The necessary condition for the ultimate toleration of very large doses is a very gradual increase in the quantities administered. Toleration can only be acquired for the last dose with a minute addition. Abrupt augmentation of the doses may, as I have ascertained, be fatal, and is accompanied by the usual symptoms of arsenical poisoning. Arsenic-eaters are in this way able to take 0.5 gr. of arsenic, or even more, and equivalent amounts of the arsenic-sulphur compound orpiment in single doses. The statement that the habitual consumption of arsenic does not make a gradual increase of the doses necessary is founded on error. Some individuals probably seek to confine the doses within certain limits or adhere to fixed doses for some time, but it is very rare for arsenic-eaters really to confess the real amount they consume.

In Germany, Austria, France, and England there are many persons who indulge in the use of arsenic. Sometimes they began taking the drug out of curiosity, sometimes after having read some book on the subject, or more frequently out of pure imitation, the cause of so many absurd actions in the world. It is taken in the belief that arsenic supplies them with a healthier appearance, as well as strength,[23] physical capacity, and endurance, which will protect them against infectious diseases. It is also taken permanently to promote sexual excitability.

It may be that arsenic-eaters copied the example of horse-dealers. Already in the sixteenth century these latter employed arsenic in order to feed worn-out horses more easily and to get them into better condition. These results, however, were not of long duration, for the horses soon became emaciated again. Even at the present day horses are not seldom doped in this manner. In the north and north-west of Styria, in the Tyrol and in Salzburg the arsenic-eaters are mainly young and old woodcutters, foresters, ostlers, etc., but also intelligent and arduous young men. This state of affairs is by no means new. I find that in 1750 a student from Halle was stated to have "intentionally accustomed himself to arsenic, which he consumed together with bacon, beginning with very small quantities. He was finally able to stand a considerable amount." In 1780 it was reported that a Tyrolese miner ate a morsel of arsenic every day in order to prolong life. The Styrian arsenic-eaters generally take the substance every week or fortnight, sometimes every second day or even daily. They begin with the "Hidrach" dose, which is the size of a millet seed, and gradually increase it to doses of the size of a pea, approximately equal to 0.1 to 0.4 gr., which they take in spirits or spread on bread or bacon. Orpiment is occasionally employed instead of arsenious acid. In some parts of Styria the consumption of arsenic is suspended during the new moon and begins again with the waxing moon in relatively small doses which are gradually increased once more to the full dose. Some refrain from drinking and eating meat or fat after having taken arsenic. The arsenic-habitués believe that it facilitates breathing during climbing. The consumption of arsenic is kept secret, especially by the female sex.

There are also male and female arsenic-eaters in the south of the United States of America, the so-called Dippers, who begin with 0.015 gr. (!) in a cup of coffee and gradually increase the doses to 0.24 gr. even twice a day. The initial difficulties such as the disagreeable eructations, together with the smell of garlic, nausea, and a feeling of heaviness in the head are easily overcome. It is stated that advanced Dippers are liable to die suddenly from slight causes, especially after the rapid withdrawal of the drug. A sudden increase is also liable to cause a serious and even fatal intoxication in arsenicists.

It is stated that snake-charmers in Persia regularly take arsenic in order to protect themselves against poisoning.

Arsenic is, however, also taken in Europe to a great extent by women and girls in certain boarding-schools where it is added to the food under the supervision of medical men. If in this case the substance is taken unconsciously and habituation and a certain craving of the cells for the irritation sets in, there are others who make use of the substance intentionally and consciously. Many ladies, including actresses, do this just as do the servants of Venus vulgivaga. A fresh complexion, a round form, smooth skin, and shining hair are attractions which lead to the use of arsenic. Hetæras who seek in this way to renew their faded charms at least justify their action by the necessity of their occupation. But when young girls take arsenic out of vainglorious imitation, and even forge medical prescriptions to obtain Fowler's solution, this certainly increasing evil should by all means be stopped. Mineral waters containing arsenic such as those of Roncegno or Levico are also consumed habitually instead of Fowler's solution.

The average daily quantity of arsenious acid which passes through the body of arsenic-eaters according to the analysis of the urine amounts to approximately 30 milligrammes, i.e. six times as much as the dose taken therapeutically. The quantities in the body, hair, marrow, etc., which sometimes becomes soluble cannot be ascertained.

It has been stated that the therapeutic application of arsenic does not develop a chronic desire for the drug because of the absence of any agreeable sensations. This is correct with respect to sufferers from skin diseases or other patients who are generally treated with such large doses in a relatively short time that their further application over a longer period would give rise to disagreeable symptoms of such a kind as to discourage all intention of continuing the drug if such were present. There are, however, cases where patients after having been cured continued to take arsenic not on account of any exciting or narcotic effects but because the prolonged use had given rise to a certain degree of habituation and they hoped to obtain the physical and æsthetic advantages mentioned above.

Habituation occurs through the adaptation of the cells, which expend both their normal and reserve energy. The fluids of the tissues do not play a part, and it is childish to assume the formation of "immunizing substances," i.e. antitoxins against arsenic, created by the organism. Medicine is so fertile in the production of absurd ideas that this is not surprising. Formerly the hypothesis was framed that the solid form in which arsenious acid is consumed excludes, or at least considerably diminishes, the possibility of intoxication because a large part of the arsenic is not resorbed and leaves the body with the fæces. It is, however, possible to become accustomed to the easily resorbable solution of the potassium salt of arsenious acid if the doses are gradually increased. Another assumption that relative immunity against arsenic is founded on a reduction or suspension of the resorption in the bowels is quite erroneous, as can be proved simply by the analysis of the urine of arsenic-eaters. The prolonged medicinal application of "Asiatic Pills," for example 3.9 gr. of arsenious acid in three months, gives rise to serious symptoms of intoxication, and on the other hand the intravenous administration of Fowler's solution even in large doses is tolerated without inconvenience.

Animals can also be habituated to tolerate large doses of arsenic. In the case of a horse the initial dose consisted of 0.36 gr. which was increased to a daily dose of 7.3 gr. within twenty-three days. The total amount the horse received was 40.46 gr. At the beginning of this treatment the animal exhibited signs of extreme vivacity and even excitation; finally diarrhœa supervened.

The most important and essential question is to ascertain whether a substance of this kind is injurious or harmless. Arsenic has recently found many defenders who had observed the good health, longevity, and flourishing appearance of a number of arsenic-eaters, and came to the conclusion that the prolonged medicinal application of arsenious acid is not accompanied by any injurious by-effects. There is no doubt that many healthy eaters of arsenic for a long time feel extremely well and that many persons who on account of some disease have taken

arsenic over a long period support it without inconvenience. It is reported that a man suffering from consumption took arsenic even in
doses of 0.1 to 0.3 gr. which he ingested and partly smoked with tobacco for six to eight weeks without any by-effects. Nevertheless this
depends upon individual sensitiveness. There are also arsenic-eaters
who after a short time suffer from the same complaints as a person
who unconsciously absorbs arsenic contained in wallpaper or objects
of daily use. Disorders of the functions set in, which become very serious and make immediate suppression of the drug necessary. A man
had consumed sodium arsenite in solution in doses of approximately 1
gr. a month for over twenty years. In the course of time gastric and
intestinal disorders occurred accompanied by disturbances of the nervous system which were similar to tabes. The colour of the skin changed
to a dirty grey, as is not rare in such cases. Nevertheless I consider the
fact that the individuals are and remain slaves to their passion as the
principal objection to chronic arsenism.

The attempt to break oneself of this drug gives rise to disagreeable
withdrawal symptoms of abstinence, such as occur with morphinism,
alcoholism, and similar vices. Especially violent gastric pains, diarrhœa,
and a state of collapse set in. The intensity of these symptoms depends upon the duration of the use of the drug and individual circumstances. An arsenic-eater who took 0.42 gr. of arsenious acid every
four to eight days and was kept well under observation suffered from
stiffness in the legs with general fatigue and craving for arsenic if he
remained abstinent for longer than a fortnight. The case of the man-
ager of an arsenic factory clearly shows that withdrawal is apt to be
fatal. He had begun with 0.18 gr., and after many years had reached
single doses of 1.38 gr. of arsenious acid in a coarse powder. When
trying to break this habit he died "of apoplexy."

MERCURY

It is not always possible to ascertain the reasons which induce man to
the habitual consumption of chemical substances of various kinds.
Metallic mercury has neither inebriating nor stimulating properties,
but it is nevertheless, as I reported some time ago,[24] taken in increasing doses of from 5 to 30 gr. at a time by Lithuanians in the district of

Memel. It is stated that boys between the ages of fourteen and sixteen start with 5 gr. The metal which has passed through the bowels is again collected in a receptacle after a due time. If the mercury is dispersed in the intestines in minute particles its vapours are liable to exercise mercurial effects. If on the other hand it passes through the intestines in a fluid mass large quantities do no harm. The Prince-Elector George of Brandenburg, who on his wedding-eve had drunk a great amount of alcohol and was therefore not conscious of his actions, emptied in a fit of thirst a whole bottle of mercury. The mercury ran through his intestines without doing him any harm whatever.

Even if the innocuousness of mercury may be understood on physical grounds, the reports of the habitual use of sublimate are incomprehensible. When the sensibility of Turkish opium-smokers to opium diminishes, and no kind of opium can be procured which supplies the desired effects, they have recourse to sublimate. They begin with 0.05 gr. (!) and gradually increase the dose so that this substance mixed with opium fully gives the expected results. Some individuals are said to have reached in this way doses of 2 gr. per day. They state that sublimate by itself is able to produce an intense feeling of well-being, but that it is especially remarkable for its capacity to sustain the narcotic effects of opium. Those who have accustomed themselves to this mercury compound combined with opium are said to take it also without opium, thereby experiencing no inconvenience. A man is said to have been observed to take a mixture of 1.2 gr. of sublimate and 3.5 gr. of opium, swallow it with apparent delight, and remain well. Sublimate is also said to be consumed habitually without opium in Peru and Bolivia in doses which must from our point of view be considered as toxic.

These reports must be doubted until more ample information is forthcoming, for it is inconceivable that sublimate should not at least exercise a local corrosive action on the intestines and in consequence rapidly prove injurious.

CONCLUSION

The chemical agents described in the preceding pages are world-wide in the good and evil results they produce. There is no doubt that a great part of these beneficial results are derived from the stimulating properties of an important group of the substances dealt with in this work which are manifested in various forms and differ in the mechanism of their effects.

The natural and internal impulses need to be artificially reinforced in the loud, harsh, and strenuous world of the present day in order to maintain biological energy at the normal standard necessary for the working of the vital functions.

The exciting or stimulating substances with which the outer world supplies us, and which have an effect on the nervous system in the manner described above, may originate from various sources. Some of them are utilized by man unconsciously, for instance in the form of the essential oils contained in the spices and vegetables which he consumes as food. It is very probable that in those cases where substances of this kind surpass the limits of toleration, become effective on a but slightly resisting organism, or are employed to excess and call forth disorders of the functions of the brain or other organs, an organic compensation will be easily established, because the use of these substances does not give rise to an eager craving for an increase of the doses, and because complete withdrawal does not occasion any disturbances.

This is not only valid for the substances of the caffeine series, but also for numerous products which are habitually chewed in many countries of the world. The greater part of them contain terpenes and are absolutely harmless. In New Zealand, for instance, the resin of the kauri pine or of a species of pittosporum is chewed, in the United States spruce gum, the resin of *pinus canadensis,* is masticated. The Tlinkit Indians use the resin of pines, the inhabitants of Siberia masticate a resinous product obtained from the bark of the larch, the Galla and Amhara incense, the Patagonians maki, a gum-resin derived from the "incense-bush," the Arabs mastix; in the United States of America and in other parts of the world the well-known chewing gum (chicle gum), the gum-resin of *achras sapota,* which is cultivated in the territory of Tuxpan in Mexico and also in Yucatan, is consumed in millions of kilogrammes. There are many other substances of a similar kind.

Narcotic substances are habitually used throughout the world to the same extent as the various kinds of stimulants, and their evil results are universal when they succeed in breaking down man's will-power with demoniacal force. The number of the unfortunate victims is increasing, and their ruin, even though there are thousands of them, is hardly of any importance compared with the cosmic process. But the fatalist who is free from hypersentimental altruism cannot shut his eyes to the fact that if the abuse of narcotic substances continues to increase at the same rate as during the last fifty years it would represent a calamity which in its consequences would concern in some way or other every one of us.

More knowledge, and especially more practical experience, seems to me indispensable in order to cope with the growing evil. Other forces than those of the police must be recruited in order to win the campaign on the one hand against the unscrupulous covetousness of merchants who are able so far to sell the worst narcotic pharmaceutical specialties and on the other against the means of satisfying the cravings of passionate drug-addicts. I have given many suggestions in this book, which is the product of the practical experience of a lifetime.

NOTES

INTRODUCTION

1. Into the heart of Nature
   No creature will ever penetrate;
   Lucky he to whom she shows
   Her outward surface.

2. ἐξ ἀρχῆς μὲν γάρ ἐνικηθὴ τὸ βραχὺ δι᾽ αὐτὴν τὴν ὀλιγότητα τω δε ἐθισμω σύμφυτον ἐγενετο.

3. L. Lewin, *Gifte und Gegengifte*, ix, Internation. Medizinischer Kongress, 1909; *Chemiker Zeitung*, 1909, No. 134; *Beiträge zur Lehre der Immunität gegen Gifte*, 3. Teile, Deutsche Medizinische Wochenschrift, 1898 and 1899.

4. L. Lewin, *Die Nebenwirkungen der Arzneimittel*, 2nd and 3rd Ed., 1899, p. 16; *Internat. Congress*, Budapest, 1909, p. 10; *Enzyklopäd. d. Medizin*, Article *Morphin*, 1910; *Die Wirkungen von Arzneimitteln und Giften auf das Auge*, 1st and 3nd Ed.

5. L. Lewin, *Untersuchungen über den Begriff der kumulativen Wirkung*, Deutsche Medizin. Wochenschrift, 1899, No. 43.

6. Santesson, *Skandinav. Archiv. für Physiologie*, vol. xxv, 1911.

7. L. Lewin, *Beiträge zur Lehre von der Immunität gegen Gifte*, Deutsche Medizin. Wochenschrift, 1898, p. 373.

8. L. Lewin *Lehrbuch der Toxikologie*, where cases of immunity against many other poisons are cited.

NARCOTIC SUBSTANCES

1. L. Lewin, *Die Nebenwirksungen der Arzneimittel*, all editions.

EUPHORICA: MENTAL SEDATIVES

1. At a later date the town of Sicyon was called Mekone, i.e., Town of Poppies, on account of the cultivation of poppies carried on there.

2. D. Lewin, *Die Gifte in der Weltgeschichte*, 1921.

3. Virgil, *Georgics*, i, 78.

4. Virgil, *Aeneid*, iv, 486; also Ovid, *Fasti*, iv, 532, 547, 661.

5. Böttiger, *Ideen*, ii, 496.

6. Silius, *De Bello Punico*, x, 353.

7. Sextus Empiricus, *Hypotyposeon*, ed. Becker: Λυσις δὲ καὶ μηκωνείον τέοσαρας ὁλύπὰς ελάμβανε.

8. Prosper Alpini, *De medicina Aegyptorum*, Lugduni Batav., 1745: *Longo tempore sic illi assuescuni, ui, mox, vel trium etiam drachmarum pondus aliqui tuto per os assumere audeani.*

9. *Confessions of an English Opium-Eater*, London, 1821.

10. Wells, *Middle Kingdom*, quoted in Lamotte, *The Opium Monopoly*, 1920. These works with their recent statistics have frequently been used in this chapter.

11. Stötzner, *Ins unerforschte Tibet*, 1924, p. 106.

12. *North China Herald*, 1910; *New York Times*, 1919; Weale in *Asia*, 1919; Macdonald, *Trade Politics and Christianity*, 1916.

13. "Kashkash," "chaščhaš" is the Arabic name for poppy, an onomatopoeic designation which represents the noise produced when shaking the ripe seeds in the capsule.

14. "I was warned that he who sleeps among the poppies falls into deep and profound dreams. On waking he retains the traces of his folly; his parents and his friends seem but shadows."

15. L. Lewin, *Berlin Klin. Wochenschrift*, 1885, p. 321.

16. L. Lewin, *Deutsche Juristenzeitung*, 1908, No. 5. See also *Die Fruchtabireibung durch Gifte*, 4th Ed., 1925.

17. *Bürgerliches Gesetzbuch*, §6.

18. L. Lewin, *Die Bestrafung der alkoholischen Trunkenheit*, Münchner Medizinische Wochenschrift, 1921, No. 46.

19. You who yearn for the month of May, pluck a bunch of violets.
    You who know you are loved, adorn yourself with the beauty of roses.
    But the child of unhappiness who desires forgetfulness
    Chooses a couch of poppies as comfort.

    When the interminable night painfully tortures,
    When he tosses in anguish on his bed of suffering;
    When everything is asleep and the ticking clock
    Hesitates in its sleepy course.

    O, he will bless you, the consolation of the martyr
    Whom an ingenious friend has brought you as cure;
    Mixed with the beverage of peace the God
    Will close the burning eyes in rest.

    The benevolent divinity approaches on his chariot
    Drawn in silence by a pair of owls; pour, oh pour
    Pearly dew that the thirsty soul be refreshed,
    Wonderful king of the realm of dreams!

    Conjure youth before his delighted spirit,
    Let him contemplate once more the radiant days of the past,
    Blow the perfumed air of May into his soul obscured by misery,
    And hope of a better future!

20. Koenig, *Berl. Klin. Wochenschrift*, 1919.

21. L. Lewin, *Berl. Klin. Wochenschrift*, 1885, p. 326.

22. The intense action of cocaine when introduced in this way may be explained by the existence of several arterial and venous systems uniting the nasal cavity with the cavities of the cranium and the corresponding lymphatic channels.

23. H. Maier, *Der Kokainismus*, 1926. The mental disturbances due to cocainism are described in this work from personal experience.

24. L. Lewin, *Die Nebenwirkungen der Arzneimittel*, 3rd ed.

25. Oppe, *Ärztl. Sachverständigen-Zeitung*, 1923, No. 1.

PHANTASTICA: HALLUCINATING SUBSTANCES

1. L. Lewin, *Deutsche Revue*, 1922, p. 57.

2. L. Lewin, *Furcht und Grauen als Unfallsursache. Obergutachten über Unfallvergiftungen*, Leipzig, 1912, p. 356.

3. L. Lewin, *Die Gifte in der Weltgeschichte*, 1920, chapter on tropeines.

4. Sahagun, *Historia general de las Cosas de Nueva España*, Lib. x, cap. xxix, §2: ". . . ellso mismos descubrieron, y usaron primero la raiz que llaman peiotl, y los que la comian y tomaban, la usaban en lugar de vino . . . y se juntaban en un llano despues de haberlo bebido, donde bailaban y cantaban de noche y de dia a su placer y esto el primer dia, porque el siguiente lloraban todos mucho . . ." Also Lib. xi, cap. vii, §1: "Hay otra yerba como tunas de la tierra, se llama peiotl, es blanca, hácase ácia la parte del norte, los que la comen ó beben ven visiones espantosas ó irrisibiles; dura esta borrachera dos ó tres dias y despues se quita; es commun manjar de los Chichimecas, pues los mantiene y da ánimo para pelear y no tener miedo, ni sed ni hambre, y dicen que los guarda de todo peligro."

5. Peyotl signifies something white and shiny, a white floccule. The cocoon of the silkworm is also called peyotl. Toca-peyotl is the spider's web.

6. Hernandez, *Historia plantar. Novae Hispaniae*, Madrid, 1721, Lib. xv, cap. xxv, p. 70.

7. Bartolom. de Alua, *Confessionario mayor y menor en lengue mexicana . . . Y platicas contra las supersticiones de idolatria . . .* 1634: "As creydo en sueños en el Peyote, Ololiuhque, en el fuego, en los Buhos, Lechusas . . ." (Ololiuhqui is a species of Datura, probably *datura meteloides*.)

8. L. Lewin, First Treatise: "Über Anhalonium Lewinii Henn.," *Archiv. für experimentelle Pathologie und Pharmakologie*, vol. xxiv, 1888, p. 401. Second Treatise: "Über Anhalonium Lewinii und andere Cacteen," *Archiv. für experimentelle Pathologie.* vol. xxxiv, 1894; *The Therapeutic Gazette*, 1888; *Pharmazeutische Zeitung*, 1895, No. 41.

9. Michaelis, *Beiträge zur vergleichenden Anatomie der Gattungen*, Echinocactus, Mamillaria und Anhalonium, 1896.

10. Heffter, *Archiv. für experim. Pathologie und Pharmakologie*, vol. xxxiv, 1894, and vol. xl, 1898.

11. L. Lewin, "Über Anhalonium Lewinii und andere giftige Kakteen," *Berichte der Deutschen Botanischen Gesellschaft*, 1894, vol. xii, Part 9.

12. ". . . una raiz que claman Peyote, á quieno dan tanta vereacion como si fuera una deidad . . ."

13. The Huichols call the god Ta-Té-awa-li.

14. This is the result of an experimental research which I suggested to Herr Jaensch.

15. Berginer, *Experimentelle Psychosen durch Mescalin*, Vortrag auf der südwestdeutschen Psychiater-Versammlung in Erlangen, 1922.

16. Majun is a saccharine preparation containing hemp to which opium, the seeds of datura, and other substances are said to be added.

17. B. Meissner in Ebert, *Reallexikon der Vorgeschichte*, vol. v, p. 117. I am indebted to Dr. John Loewenthal for this information.

18. L. Lewin, *Lehrbuch der Toxicologie*, 2nd ed., p. 379.

19. Arnoldi Abbatis Lubecensis, *Chronica Slavorum*, l. iii, c. xxxvii, p. 349; l. vii, c. x, p. 523: ". . . eis cultros quasi ad hoc negotium sacratos, administrat, et tunc poculos eos quodam, quo in ecstasin vel amentiam rapiantur, inebriat et eis magicis suis quaedam somnia phantastica, gaudiis et deliciis, imo nugis plena, ostendit . . ."

20. L. Lewin, *Die Gifte in der Weltgeschichte*, 1920, p. 207.

21. Artbauer, *Rifpiraten*, 1911.

22. According to Hügel, not only the comon people but also the Brahmins smoke the dried blossoms.

23. L. Lewin, *Die Gifte in der Weltgeschichte*, Berlin, 1920.

24. Ibid.

25. L. Lewin, *Die Gifte in der Weltgeschichte*, 1920, p. 4.

26. See p. 116.

27. Acacia leaves are said to be added to pituri.

28. Reinberg, *Journale de la Société des Américanistes de Paris*, t. xiii, p. 25, 1921. The statements about curare which are borrowed from medical literature have nothing in common with the substance in question.

29. See section on *Agaricus muscarius*, pp. 102–107.

INEBRIANTIA

1. Erman-Ranke, *Agypten*, 2nd ed., p. 288.

2. Erman-Ranke, loc. cit.

3. Soma or homa is said to be *periploca aphylla, sarcostemma brevistigma, setaria glauca, ephedra vulgaris* and other plants. But none of these plants is able to give rise to such effects as have been attributed to soma.

4. A beverage prepared from this plant is called *kiwa* in the south of the Gran Chaco.

5. Spirits obtained from molasses are probably also called *samshu*.

6. Ambroise, Paré, *Opera*, p. 1154.

7. Bobba u. Mauro, *Alpine Schriften des Priesters Achille Ratti*, 1925, p. 44.

8. Montaigne, *Essays*, Book ii, chap. 2

9. Balusius, *Capitularia regum Francorum*, Venetiis, 1722, pp. 257, 177, 782.

10. ". . . a communione statuimus submovendum aut corporali subdendum esse supplicio."

11. L. Lewin, *Die Restrafung der alkoholischen Trunkenheit* (Kritik des Strafgesetzentwurfes von 1919), Münchn. Med. Wochenschrift, 1921, No. 45.

12. L. Lewin, *Die Nebenwirkungen der Arzneimittel*, 1893, p. 67; 1899, p. 51.

13. L. Lewin, *Die Nebenwirkungen der Arzneimittel*, 1893, etc., chapter on Inhalations-Anästhetika.

HYPNOTICA: SOPORIFICS

1. L. Lewin, *Die Nebenwirkungen der Arzneimittel*, 3rd ed.

2. L. Lewin, *Über* Piper Methysticum (*Kawa-Kawa*). Monographie, Berlin, 1886. *Berlin. klin. Wochenschrift*, 1886, No. 1. A *Lecture on Piper Methysticum*, Detroit, 1886.

EXCITANTIA

1. L. Lewin, *Über Areca Catechu, Chavica Betle und das Betelkauen*. Eine Monographie, Stuttgart, 1889.

2. Young nuts are stated to contain less arecoline than older ones.

3. In Yemen only an infusion of the husks of coffee is consumed.

4. Leonharti Rauwolfen, *Aigentliche Beschreibung der Raisz in die Morgenländer*, 1582, p. 102.

5. Carl Ritter, *Vergleichende Erdkunde von Arabien*, vol. ii, p. 579.

6. Steindorff, *Durch die Lybische Wuste*, 1904, p. 88.

7. Silvestre de Sacy, *Chrestomathie arabe*, vol. i, p. 439.

8. Redi, *Bacco in Toscana*, Ditirambo, Napoli, 1742, p. 6.

9. Virchow, *Nahrungs- und Genussmittel*, 1868.

10. L. Lewin, *Die Nebenwirkungen der Arzneimittel*, 3rd ed.

11. L. Lewin, *Die Nebenwirkungen der Arzneimittel*, all editions.

12. Lyre, murmur sweetly

    Hardly touched by light fingers!

    You sing of the most delicate thing

    The world contains.

    It is in India, the land of mystery,

    Where spring always reigns.

    Where tea, itself a myth.

    Lives and loves and flourishes.

    Vom leichten Finger kaum geregt!

    Ihr tönet zu des Zärtsten Preise,

    Des Zäctsten, was die Erde hegt.

    In Indiens mythischem Gebiete,

    Wo Frühling ewig sich ernent,

    O Tee, du selber eine Mythe,

    Verlebst du deine Blütenzeit.

13. These tables probably have little claim to accuracy at the present time.

14. "Joudz ez-zenj is a fruit of the size of an apple, somewhat elongated, wrinkled and angular. It contains seeds similar to cardamoms which are

flat (round), brown (red) and have an aromatic odour. They are brought from the mountainous territory of the Berbers and applied against flatulent colic."

15. The "Cola vera" of Herr Schumann does not exist. The many "new" species of kola have been discovered without their chemical properties being examined. I have pointed out that we cannot consider a morphologic examination sufficient and decisive in this respect. (L. Lewin, *Berichte der Deutschen Botanischen Gesellschaft*, 1894, Heft 9.)

16. Kolanine or kola-red, an amorphous powder insoluble in water, is said to be a glucosid. This has in the meantime been rejected and no chemical or pharmaco-dynamic effects are stated to appear. A so-called Tanno-glucosid which is said to split into caffeine, glucose, and kola-red caffeine is stated to be a mixture of kolatin and caffeine.

17. The recent opinion that the active principle (mattein) is not identical with caffeine must be rejected. But it is possible that other purine bases are contained in maté beside caffeine.

18. It has been reported that an infusion containing alcohol obtained through fermentation is also drunk. *Eryngium aquaticum* or *lobelia inflata* are said to be added to the infusion.

19. *Guarana* (uarana) signifies a creeping plant in the language of the Tupis.

20. L. Lewin, *Die Gifte in der Weltgeschichte*, 1920.

21. L. Lewin, *Die Nebenwirkungen der Arzneimittel*, 2nd and 3rd eds., and L. Lewin in Lewin and Guillery, *Die Wirkungen von Arzneimitteln und Giften auf das Auge*, 2nd ed., 1907, Bd. I.

22. L. Lewin, *Die Nebenwirkungen der Arzneimittel*, 2nd and 3rd eds.

23. It has been found that young growing rabbits fed daily with 1/2000 gr. of arsenious acid developed physically to a greater degree than those not so treated. This effect of the arsenic irritation on the tissues, however, is only temporary, and is soon succeeded by contrary results. This irritating effect, which is liable to lead to an augmentation of growth and cell-formation, is far less efficacious in adult animals. The results of these experimental investigations throw no light on the consumption of arsenic by man.

24. L. Lewin, *Über eigentümliche Quecksilberanwendungen*, Berlin. klin. Wochenschrift, 1899, No. 13.

INDEX